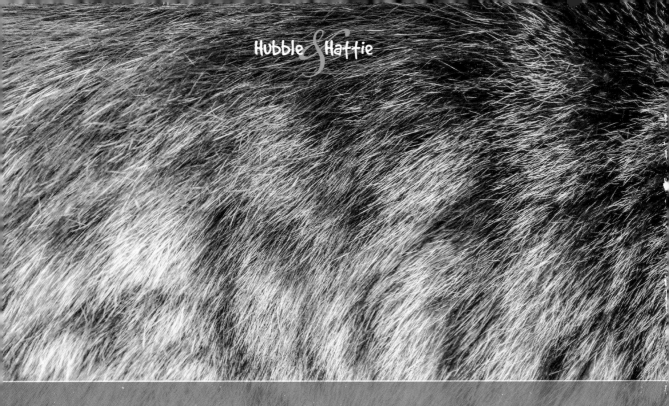

Hubble & Hattie

The Complete Book of
CAT & DOG HEALTH

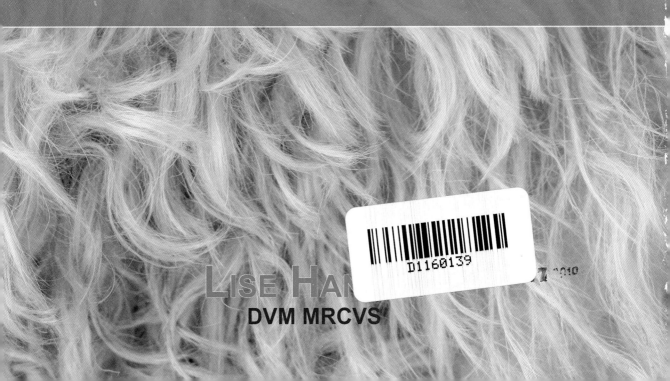

LISE HANSEN
DVM MRCVS

The Hubble & Hattie imprint was launched in 2009 and is named in memory of two very special Westies owned by Veloce's proprietors. Since the first book, many more have been added to the list, all with the same underlying objective: to be of real benefit to the species they cover, at the same time promoting compassion, understanding and respect between all animals (including human ones!)

Hubble & Hattie is the home of a range of books that cover all-things animal, produced to the same high quality of content and presentation as our motoring books, and offering the same great value for money.

More great Hubble & Hattie books!
Among the Wolves: Memoirs of a wolf handler (Shelbourne)
Animal Grief: How animals mourn (Alderton)
Babies, kids and dogs – creating a safe and harmonious relationship (Fallon & Davenport)
Because this is our home ... the story of a cat's progress (Bowes)
Bonds – Capturing the special relationship that dogs share with their people (Cukuraite & Pais)
Camper vans, ex-pats & Spanish Hounds: from road trip to rescue – the strays of Spain (Coates & Morris)
Canine aggression – how kindness and compassion saved Calgacus (McLennan)
Cat and Dog Health, The Complete Book of (Hansen)
Cat Speak: recognising & understanding behaviour (Rauth-Widmann)
Charlie – The dog who came in from the wild (Tenzin-Dolma)
Clever dog! Life lessons from the world's most successful animal (O'Meara)
Complete Dog Massage Manual, The – Gentle Dog Care (Robertson)
Confessions of a veterinary nurse: paws, claws and puppy dog tails (Ison)
Detector Dog – A Talking Dogs Scentwork Manual (Mackinnon)
Dieting with my dog: one busy life, two full figures ... and unconditional love (Frezon)
Dinner with Rover: delicious, nutritious meals for you and your dog to share (Paton-Ayre)
Dog Cookies: healthy, allergen-free treat recipes for your dog (Schöps)
Dog-friendly gardening: creating a safe haven for you and your dog (Bush)
Dog Games – stimulating play to entertain your dog and you (Blenski)
Dog Relax – relaxed dogs, relaxed owners (Pilguj)
Dog Speak: recognising & understanding behaviour (Blenski)
Dogs just wanna have Fun! Picture this: dogs at play (Murphy)
Dogs on Wheels: travelling with your canine companion (Mort)
Emergency First Aid for dogs: at home and away Revised Edition (Bucksch)
Exercising your puppy: a gentle & natural approach – Gentle Dog Care (Robertson & Pope)
For the love of Scout: promises to a small dog (Ison)
Fun and Games for Cats (Seidl)
Gods, ghosts, and black dogs – the fascinating folklore and mythology of dogs (Coren)
Helping minds meet – skills for a better life with your dog (Zulch & Mills)
Home alone – and happy! Essential life skills for preventing separation anxiety in dogs and puppies (Mallatratt)
Know Your Dog – The guide to a beautiful relationship (Birmelin)
Letting in the dog: opening hearts and minds to a deeper understanding (Blocker)
Life skills for puppies – laying the foundation for a loving, lasting relationship (Zuch & Mills)
Lily: One in a million! A miracle of survival (Hamilton)
Living with an Older Dog – Gentle Dog Care (Alderton & Hall)
Miaow! Cats really are nicer than people! (Moore)
Mike&Scrabble – A guide to training your new Human (Dicks & Scrabble)
Mike&Scrabble Too – Further tips on training your Human (Dicks & Scrabble)
My cat has arthritis – but lives life to the full! (Carrick)

My dog has arthritis – but lives life to the full! (Carrick)
My dog has cruciate ligament injury – but lives life to the full! (Haüsler & Friedrich)
My dog has epilepsy – but lives life to the full! (Carrick)
My dog has hip dysplasia – but lives life to the full! (Haüsler & Friedrich)
My dog is blind – but lives life to the full! (Horsky)
My dog is deaf – but lives life to the full! (Willms)
My Dog, my Friend: heart-warming tales of canine companionship from celebrities and other extraordinary people (Gordon)
Office dogs: The Manual (Rousseau)
One Minute Cat Manager: sixty seconds to feline Shangri-la (Young)
Ollie and Nina and ... daft doggy doings! (Sullivan)
No walks? No worries! Maintaining wellbeing in dogs on restricted exercise (Ryan & Zulch)
Partners – Everyday working dogs being heroes every day (Walton)
Puppy called Wolfie – a passion for free will teaching (Gregory)
Smellorama – nose games for dogs (Theby)
Supposedly enlightened person's guide to raising a dog (Young & Tenzin-Dolma)
Swim to recovery: canine hydrotherapy healing – Gentle Dog Care (Wong)
Tale of two horses – a passion for free will teaching (Gregory)
Tara – the terrier who sailed around the world (Forrester)
Truth about Wolves and Dogs, The: dispelling the myths of dog training (Shelbourne)
Unleashing the healing power of animals: True stories about therapy animals – and what they do for us (Preece-Kelly)
Waggy Tails & Wheelchairs (Epp)
Walking the dog: motorway walks for drivers & dogs revised edition (Rees)
When man meets dog – what a difference a dog makes (Blazina)
Wildlife photography – saving my life one frame at a time (Williams)
Winston ... the dog who changed my life (Klute)
Wonderful walks from dog-friendly campsites throughout the UK (Chelmicka)
Worzel Wooface: For the love of Worzel (Pickles)
Worzel Wooface: The quite very actual adventures of (Pickles)
Worzel Wooface: The quite very actual Terribibble Twos (Pickles)
Worzel Wooface: Three quite very actual cheers for (Pickles)
You and Your Border Terrier – The Essential Guide (Alderton)
You and Your Cockapoo – The Essential Guide (Alderton)
Your dog and you – understanding the canine psyche (Garratt)

Hubble & Hattie Kids!
Fierce Grey Mouse (Bourgonje)
Indigo Warrios: The Adventure Begins! (Moore)
Lucky, Lucky Leaf, The: A Horace & Nim story (Bourgonje & Hoskins)
Little house that didn't have a home, The (Sullivan & Burke)
Lily and the Little Lost Doggie, The Adventures of (Hamilton)
My Grandad can draw anything ... but he can't draw hands! (Sullivan & Burke)
Positive Thinking for Piglets: A Horace & Nim story (Bourgonje & Hoskins)
Wandering Wildebeest, The (Coleman & Slater)
Worzel goes for a walk! Will you come too? (Pickles & Bourgonje)
Worzel says hello! Will you be my friend? (Pickles & Bourgonje)

www.hubbleandhattie.com

First published in October 2019 by Veloce Publishing Limited, Veloce House, Parkway Farm Business Park, Middle Farm Way, Poundbury, Dorchester, Dorset, DT1 3AR, England. Tel 01305 260068/fax 01305 250479/e-mail info@hubbleandhattie.com/web www.hubbleandhattie.com. ISBN: 978-1-787114-15-9 UPC: 6-36847-01415-5.
Readers with ideas for books about animals, or animal-related topics, are invited to write to the editorial director of Veloce Publishing at the above address. British Library Cataloguing in Publication Data - A catalogue record for this book is available from the British Library. Typesetting, design and page make-up all by Veloce Publishing Ltd on Apple Mac. Printed and bound in India by Parkson Graphics PVT Ltd

A comment on language

I disagree fundamentally with the notion that we can ever really own another living being, and so I try to avoid the term 'owner,' using instead 'carer.'

In places, though, this has felt too affected and I have used owner for lack of a better alternative. I happily refer to your dog the way I would your father, implying not ownership, but merely referring to a member of your family.

In an attempt to save ink and time, throughout I have chosen to refer to animals as 'he' and 'him', and to vets as 'she' and 'her.' I hope you'll bear with me.

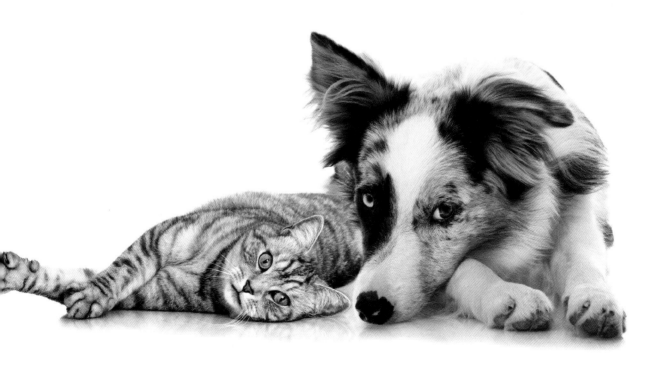

Contents

Foreword

by Andrew Prentis

After nearly 40 years in the veterinary world in private practice, charity clinics, teaching at university, and in development work overseas, I have seen quite a few animals and quite a few different ways of managing animal health and disease.

I have seen many, many animals get better, and equally, a fair number where diet, neutering, vaccination or medication have had adverse effects on their overall health. And even some where their continuing to thrive seems to be more a result of luck and strong genes than good judgement on the part of their carers.

Medicine is both a science and an art, and is not as neatly defined and circumscribed as many of its practitioners would like. Often finding myself in front of keen and highly educated veterinary students eager for pearls of wisdom from an old hand, I have sometimes struggled to know where to start, because a lot of what I have had to say runs contrary to conventional thinking in veterinary practice.

So, in a slightly flippant mood, I found myself writing 'The Ten Commandments of Veterinary Practice' with some of those vet students in mind. It is a distillation of my experience; an attempt to set down in writing some of the things that I felt to be true and useful to vets in practice: principles that I have tried to incorporate into my clinical work and to communicate to the vets and students around me. At the end of this foreword you'll find a version adapted for pet owners.

It was only a few weeks after this that I found myself being asked to read Lise's book, and I have to say that I agree with almost every word she has to say.

Lise talks about her subject not only with a real wealth of knowledge and experience, but also with warmth, humour, and an obvious and deep concern for the health of her patients. She is a very practical and pragmatic person who applies the principles she has researched and studied, and has seen to work time and time again. It's all here, so please read on.

Lise is right to suggest that we should take a closer look at some of the protocols so widely used for pet neutering, parasite control, diet and vaccination. Given what we now know about the side effects of neutering, the dangers of overuse of pesticides, the damage caused by highly processed 'junk' food, and the ease with which we can check an animal's antibody levels before revaccinating, it's fair to ask whether these protocols are really evidence-based or more eminence-based (as in 'it's what we were taught at vet school years ago').

The concept of holistic health care, and homeopathy in particular, is very controversial in the veterinary world at the moment. Clinicians like Lise are understandably a little tired of continually being challenged to justify their clinical choices when, in her words, "I see the 'incurable' being cured on a daily basis, and I'm a little tired of having to fight my corner all the time. I just want to get on with my work."

If Lise considers the writing of this book to be 'just getting on with my work,' I am in awe of her achievement.

I am not alone in having seen the cases and heard firsthand from clients about dramatic health improvements that have resulted from – or at least coincided with – the adoption of a more appropriate diet, or the application of forms of holistic medicine. I am not a homeopath, nor an acupuncturist or osteopath, but there is no doubt in my mind that holistic health care has its place alongside what we currently refer to as conventional medicine.

There are many who would like to follow Lise's approach, and I wholeheartedly commend this book to them, as it clearly helps to set the record straight: whether or not you accept that homeopathy or herbs have a role, we should be paying attention to the information now available to us, and be prepared to rethink some of the basics of how we care for our animal companions.

Lise presents here a wealth of up-to-date information, evidence and advice that I hope will help persuade animal carers – and their vets – that it's time to look again at animal health, and not just blindly follow the commercial interests of 'big pharma.' With her help and guidance, there is a much brighter future ahead for the animals in our care.

The Ten Polite Suggestions for Veterinary Practice, for pet owners everywhere

1   Seek out vets who offer longer consultations. If your vet is seeing more than 12 patients a day, every day, she might be struggling to find the time to practice really good medicine, or indeed, give you good value for money. It takes a while to get a proper history and put all the information in the right order. It may help make the diagnosis, but it does take time, so give her the space to do the work that is in front of you both

2   Choose vets who are kind to your pets, and always spend a bit of time noodling with them. It's much less fun if they don't

3   Ask if they really need to inject everything. Your pets don't like it, and it rarely makes any significant difference to how quickly the medicines start to work

4   Wherever possible, encourage your vet to test before treatment. This doesn't only apply to bacterial infections and antibiotics – it's equally important for parasitic disease and vaccination programmes, so help them make it a habit. Titre test before vaccinating for Distemper, Hepatitis and Parvovirus in dogs, and consider it for Panleucopenia in cats

5   Don't vaccinate against diseases that your pets are extremely unlikely to have any contact with

6   Don't treat parasitic diseases that aren't there. Help your vet to risk-assess your

pet's lifestyle, and find out what the local disease incidence is: you can do this by calling around some of the other local practices and simply asking them. In adult animals routinely request faecal worm egg counts before giving any parasite treatments. Develop prevention or treatment regimes accordingly, and don't overtreat

7 Accept that most pets have a fully functioning immune system and will get better anyway. An important part of your vet's job is to figure out which ones are serious and need action now, and which ones can be given time ... and there's a real skill in that. Sometimes 'I don't think we need to do anything else right now' or 'I think it's safe to wait and see what happens overnight' is enough. 'I don't know' is okay, too, providing there's a plan

8 Be open-minded about other systems of medicine. Some of their practitioners and clients are every bit as clever, educated and discerning as you are, and the results they report at least merit some attention. It is possible that they may have something to contribute to our understanding of medicine and how the body works, and it is also possible that they may be having successes where conventional medicine struggles

9 Neutering an animal is never an entirely benign procedure. Weigh up the real data on behavioural change, incidence of neoplasia, thyroid disease and skeletal abnormalities before making any decision. It's not just about convenience, incontinence and weight gain

10 Be prepared to at least give raw feeding a try. Don't be afraid to involve your vet in the diet discussion: it may not be for everyone, but you'll find that many pets will love it and thrive on it

Andrew Prentis MRCVS
The Hyde Park Veterinary Centre
London

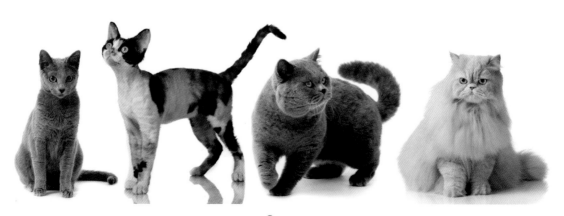

Introduction

Many dogs and cats live long and healthy lives without needing treatment of any kind: a combination, probably, of good care, good genes and good luck. Most animals, however, are not quite as blessed, and will at some point in their life become ill and have to visit a vet. Some of these recover completely, but after 25 years as a veterinary surgeon, I am deeply aware that far, far too many don't. It was these dogs and cats who live with constant or recurring health problems, these 'repeat offenders' who return to the vet year in and year out with the same chronic problem, who, early in my veterinary career, made me question whether we could do things differently. The truth is that there is so much we can do better.

If you've ever known a dog or cat who is continually in and out of veterinary clinics, then you know what I'm talking about.

This book is a companion for everybody with a love for animals and an interest in their health and wellbeing. Whether you share your life with a healthy animal, or one who suffers from a chronic condition, this book will help you make sense of recent changes in expert veterinary advice.

The book is in three parts –

The first part covers all of the issues that face carers trying to provide their animal with a healthy lifestyle, and includes the latest expert advice on vaccination and neutering.

The second part introduces holistic veterinary healthcare, and describes the major holistic treatment methods.

The final part consists of an overview of a number of common health problems. This section includes lots of practical advice on how you can supplement and support the treatment your vet is offering.

It is my sincere hope that this book will help prevent and alleviate illness for the animals who share and enrich our lives. I hope that it will enable you to care for the animal in your life in a way that feels right to you.

Lise Hansen DVM MRCVS CertIAVH
PCH
Veterinary Surgeon and Classical
Homeopath

PART ONE
A healthy life

What is a healthy life for a cat or a dog?

Being healthy means so much more than simply not being ill. Optimal health demands a lifestyle that suits the mental, emotional and physical needs of the individual. Exercise, meaningful social interaction and mental stimulation are all required for natural development.

It is worth remembering that the very fact that we keep dogs and cats as pets means that we take away their power and ability to choose for themselves, even in adulthood. Some will argue that the cat who is kept indoors, and never in his life catches a mouse, or the dog who is left home alone for ten hours a day, and is perhaps rarely let off the lead on walks, can never be a fulfilled and balanced individual.

I take the view that, by the very act of keeping animals, we take on full responsibility for their wellbeing, and are therefore obligated to stay well informed, and do our utmost to make the best choices on their behalf.

I believe that both humans and animals benefit hugely from sharing our lives, and that we have come a long way in recent years in terms of understanding and respecting both the behavioural and physical needs of dogs and cats.

The first part of this book discusses the lifestyle choices that we must make on behalf of the animals in our care.

The beginning

Arrival of your puppy or kitten

A whole lifetime. About 15 years – a little less for a dog; perhaps a little longer for a cat. That's no small commitment. Not only are we talking about their lives, but their contribution to our lives, which is indescribable. It goes without saying that we should do everything in our power to start off on the right foot, laying the foundation for a harmonious life together.

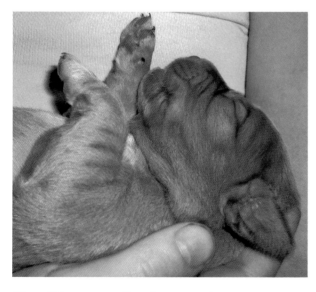

The all-important first four months

The most important character-forming period of a dog's life is the first 16 weeks. During these first few months of life, the puppy is

Three weeks to three months: the important window

The risk of an unvaccinated puppy catching a potentially fatal contagious disease is infinitesimally smaller than the risk of a potentially fatal behavioural problem arising from lack of proper socialisation. Ergo, puppies need to be out in the world, learning not to be fearful, and learning how to interact. Missing out on this is the single biggest risk, not only to their (and your) quality of life, but also to their longevity. Vaccinated or not, never isolate a puppy.

open to new experiences in a unique way, and this is when the foundation for good mental health is established.

Between the age of three weeks and three to four months, a puppy's brain is uniquely malleable and primed to learn about the world. This is when he learns about relating to humans, other dogs, and all the sounds and sights around him. It's as though he observes everything he meets – sounds, experiences, objects – and simply concludes, 'Okay, that exists and is fine. I'll remember that.'

At 16 weeks (sometimes earlier), something fundamental happens to the puppy's brain, and therefore to his approach to the world: it's as though the brain, to some degree, closes down or freezes. Everything experienced *before* this age is stored and remembered forever as being okay, but things experienced for the first time *after* this age are more likely to be met with fear, and the attitude, 'I know what's safe in the world, and I don't know this.' From the age of three weeks to three months, new sounds, sights and experiences are nothing to be feared, but after this age, the response is likely to be much more sceptical, especially in a puppy who is not already used to constantly taking in and accepting new aspects of an ever-expanding world. Fear is at the root of most aggressive behaviour in dogs, which is why it is simply not possible to exaggerate the lasting effect of the first three to four months of life on a dog's character – in fact, on his entire life.

His life before you

The period from when the puppy first opens his eyes (when he is nearly two weeks old) until he is around 16 weeks old is the all-important period of socialisation. During these early months, the brain is uniquely malleable and open to new impressions, and most reasonably positive new experiences will be accepted immediately. By contrast, experiences that are met for the first time later in life can be much harder to accept, and may require lengthy training.

Don't waste this golden period, and be aware that at least half of it has already passed by the time you take home your new family member: your puppy or kitten is formed by their experiences long before they move in with you. They notice how their mother reacts to people, to other animals, to approaching strangers, to noises, and so on. Everything will be easier (not to mention that you will be supporting good breeding practices rather than funding puppy farming) if you choose a well-stimulated, bold, curious and lively puppy or

kitten instead of the timid one, who is scared of life and far too easily overwhelmed because he has spent his first months tucked away in a kennel with only his mother and siblings. It is my opinion that a 'kitchen-floor litter' has the very best start in life, growing up amidst the hustle and bustle of everyday human activity, being regularly handled and picked up for cuddles and kisses, exposed to children with high voices and quick movements, men with deep voices, and doors opening, cupboards closing, phones ringing, and Hoovers hoovering.

Studies have shown that puppies who are handled by humans daily from the age of only a few days retain closer bonds to people for the rest of their lives, and can be distinguished from their littermates who lacked these very early experiences. Isn't that something? And doesn't it make it all the more worthwhile to put in the effort from the outset and make sure you find the right breeder?

Seeing is believing

Always visit the litter while the puppies or kittens are still with their mother. Ideally, go long before they are even old enough to leave her. Some breeders don't allow visits during the first month, as this can introduce unfamiliar germs and generally disturb the nursing

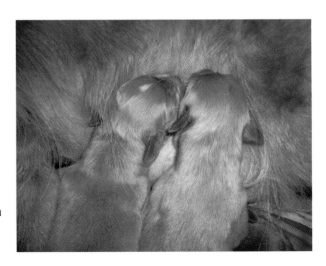

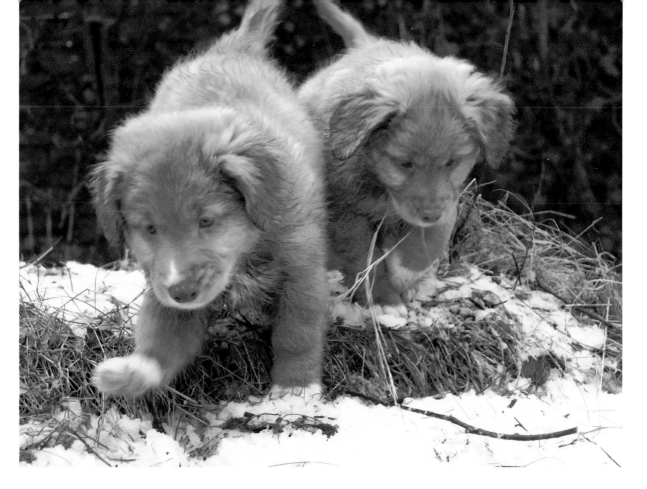

mother. That's fine. Once the puppies are five weeks old, however, you should be able to visit.

Your first visit is simply to get an impression of the place. You want to meet the breeder, see where the puppies are growing up, and see the mother. All puppies are irresistible to anyone in possession of a heart, so go ahead and delight over them, but remember that the mother will give you a much better impression of what kind of dog you may be getting. If the breeder swiftly removes her to let you focus on the puppies, ask to spend some time with her, too. Is she friendly and approachable, or is she shy and reserved, or very protective of the puppies? Buyers who don't see at least one of the puppy's parents are at higher risk of choosing a dog who will require professional help for behavioural problems. This may simply reflect the fact that experienced dog people will always insist on

meeting the parents, or it could indicate that buyers who did meet the parents took home puppies that were actually more mentally stable. Of course, one explanation doesn't rule out the other; both could be true. Just remember the bottom line: don't take the puppy if you can't meet the mother.

If you set out to visit a litter of eight-week-old puppies for the first time, expecting to return home with a new family member, it requires almost superhuman willpower to back out, even if your alarm bells start to ring during the visit. It's much better to go for the first time knowing that this is just a visit (a scouting mission, if you like). Ideally, visit the litter more than once, and visit more than one litter. You can always return if you liked what you saw, but I do recommend that you always leave empty-handed after the first visit. Go home and sleep on it.

Faced with a litter that is obviously

growing up in less-than-ideal circumstances, it is a natural urge to want to rescue at least one of the puppies. Believe me, I do understand the temptation to sweep up the scared puppy in front of you and give him a better life, but know that, by doing so, you are supporting the puppy-farming industry, and ensuring that many more puppies will be raised in similar conditions. We can only stop bad breeding by not buying the puppies. If, on the other hand, you buy from an informed and loving breeder who raises mentally and physically healthy puppies, you will not only ensure that you bring the best possible dog into your family but will also support responsible breeding in the future.

Ready or not?

Many countries have legislation that stipulates the earliest time that a puppy can legally be removed from his mother and put up for sale. Most agree on eight weeks as the magic number.

For some reason, there are fewer laws in place to protect kittens. Most experts agree that, while eight weeks is ideal for a puppy, it is too early for a kitten to be separated from his mother and littermates. At eight weeks, he may be eating solids, but he is still busy learning how to be a cat. The discussion is ongoing as to whether 12, 13 or even 14 weeks or more is the optimal age for a kitten to leave his mother and move to a new home.

Don't waste precious time

True, some breeds are a bit slower to mature, so you won't hear me say that there is never a situation where it may be in the puppy's best interest to stay with his mother until he is nine or even ten weeks old. As a rule, though, these are precious weeks indeed, and, once he has reached eight weeks, you really want him home so that you can introduce him to his new life, and take charge of the socialisation process. If the puppy you are looking at will

be four months old before your holiday plans or other commitments allow you to pick him up, I strongly recommend that you reconsider. Maybe another puppy will suit you better. Maybe next year the timing will be right.

The big day

When the big day finally arrives, and you set off to bring home your new family member, be prepared to cancel if he is not well. You should postpone the pickup at any sign of acute illness (perhaps caused by an ill-timed first vaccination; see page 51). If it's only a harmless bug and he's fine after three days, get him then, but if it turns out to be the first sign of chronic problems, you will want to find out what it is before you take him on. Puppies and kittens must be healthy when they leave their mothers and move into their permanent homes.

Time to meet the world

The breeder has done her part; now it's time for you to take charge of the socialisation process. The importance of proper socialisation cannot be exaggerated. The first three to four months of a puppy's life will shape the next ten to 15 years, and the time and effort you invest at this stage will be amply repaid by the sociable and well-functioning adult dog who will share your life for years to come.

Mad world

Make sure that your puppy gets out and about: goes on car rides, and walks on pavements, bridges, gravel and grass. Says hello to other animals of all ages, shapes and sizes. Meets people with crutches, caps and canes. Encounters scooters, wheelchairs, containers, tarpaulins, bells and whistles. Experiences thunder, rain, umbrellas, brooms, Hoovers, clothes racks and shopping trolleys. Learns

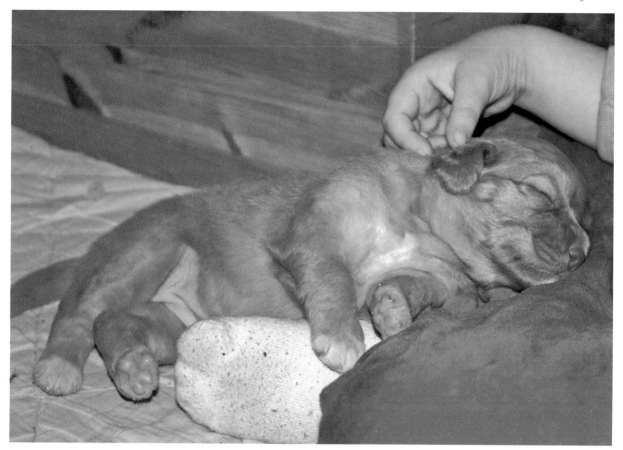

about bicycles, trains, buses, wheelbarrows and jet planes. Now is the time for him to experience it all. All of these things can be very scary if met for the first time later in life, and, as already mentioned, by the time your puppy is approaching his four-month birthday, it is already getting late.

There are CDs and online videos that introduce a variety of noises (thunder, fireworks) for exactly this purpose. I know great breeders who play these while the tiny puppies are nursing.

Keep it positive

Never deliberately frighten your puppy, as this will have the exact opposite effect to what you are trying to achieve. If a person, sound or object doesn't seem safe to him, don't

pull or carry him to it, or try to cajole him into going closer. Simply stay at a reasonably safe distance and remain calm and unaffected. Take your time, ignore him, and see if he doesn't eventually get bored and curious enough to venture forward himself. If so, you can follow with measured praise and encouragement.

Just as it's important to tick off the positive encounters on the 'okay' list, it's also important not to overwhelm or frighten your puppy with a bad experience that will be remembered forever. You are collecting positive experiences. Keep a constant eye on your puppy's reactions and stop before he becomes overwhelmed. He should absolutely meet and greet dogs of both sexes and all breeds, sizes and ages, but first quickly check with the owner to ensure that their dog is friendly, and not inclined to eat puppies for breakfast.

A small dog is still a dog

As soon as your puppy has had a week or so to settle into his new home, it is time to start puppy classes. This is primarily a place for him to practice socialising, and for you to have access to and learn from a competent dog trainer.

It is my experience that owners of large-breed puppies are very aware of the importance of socialising and training, whereas some feel that this is less important in the case of small dogs. After all, they require less exercise, and can be entertained in the garden or on a lead, and if there is trouble, you can just pick them up, right? Wrong. Optimal socialisation is equally important for a small-breed puppy. The world can easily become a scary and overwhelming place when everyone is much bigger than you. A small dog is a dog, too, and needs to be able to conduct himself – which is not to say that you shouldn't be there to protect him if he needs help.

A retractable lead gives neither freedom nor control

Let your puppy run free every day. I am not a fan of retractable dog leads, and they are in no way a substitute for letting your dog run free. Never use a retractable lead on pavements, on paths, in parks or any place where you meet other people or animals. It is unnecessary and unsafe. He must have recall, and he must have time off the lead.

By all means, use a retractable lead if you are walking far from traffic and unlikely to meet anyone. Maybe your dog is still being trained, maybe your bitch is on heat or perhaps the terrain is unsafe. It is only a tool, and sometimes it may serve a purpose, so I will not blame the tool but only the way that it is easily misunderstood and misused as a

substitute for training and proper control. It is easy to regard a retractable lead as a way to allow your dog some space while still retaining control when, in fact, it achieves neither. It is not a substitute for free play, and it gives only an illusion of control, which is why it is so dangerous. I have known more than one dog who was run over by a car while the owner was still holding the other end of the lead. What are you going to do when your dog spots his best friend (or his arch enemy – perhaps in the form of a squirrel) on the opposite pavement, and dives into traffic? Even if you possess ninja-like reflexes and lock the mechanism before he is halfway across the street, you still have a dog at the end of a very long, thin line that will inflict severe rope burn if you grab and pull on the line itself. And what about the day when the mechanism breaks, as they all do at some point?

Use a proper lead in situations when you need a lead (such as anywhere near traffic), and find a safe space to let him off the lead to run and play every day.

Puppy time

Having a puppy in the house is much like having a baby, the main difference being that, as with everything else in a dog's life, it is a much shorter phase. Your new puppy will demand 100% of your time and attention for the first few weeks only. Don't expect to get a full night's sleep; his bladder is still small, and he'll most likely stir in the night and need you to take him out to pee. Set aside a holiday for Project Puppy. If he has your full attention, it will take only two to three weeks to get him fully house-trained and settled.

Home alone

As you begin your second week together, and your puppy seems to have forgotten already that he didn't always live in this house with this lovely human family, it is time to begin leaving him alone for ten minutes at a time.

Almost all the dogs that I have been asked to treat for separation anxiety (see the section on behavioural problems, page 204) belonged to people who forgot to include home-alone training, because there was simply no urgent need to leave the puppy.

Of course, it is possible to teach a dog of any age to be home alone, but if you include it in his early training, it will come much more easily. Even if you are on maternity leave, are a pensioner, work from home or, for any other reason, can supply round-the-clock company for your puppy, don't. He needs to learn (long before he is four months old, remember?) that humans come and go, and that this is perfectly fine. It is all a part of the natural way of things; it's how the world works.

Basic trust
The world is a safe and friendly place, and you are at its centre, emanating all that is good. If this is your pup's worldview, bravo – you have succeeded, and you and your puppy are well on your way. The old-school approach (popular around the turn of the millennium), based on the assumption that your puppy was planning world domination unless you kept him in his place at all times, has very much been abandoned and replaced by the realisation that, much like everyone else, puppies just want to feel good. Reward desirable behaviour, and this is what you'll get. Your puppy doesn't want to be your boss; he just wants to feel good right now, and is therefore likely to repeat the behaviour that brings treats, games and praise.

'Dominance' is no longer considered a relevant concept; 'positive reinforcement' is the name of the game. Be calm, loving and supportive. You are always on his side. You are there to guide him and to help him when he needs help. The last thing you want is for your puppy to lose trust or even become scared of you. It makes no more sense to scold a puppy who peed on the floor than it

does to scold a baby for soiling her nappy. As soon as he understands what is expected of him, he will cooperate. Step by step, introduce him to the world and show him his place in it. Take him everywhere from day one, but don't overwhelm or frighten him. Keep it positive.

The piranha phase
All puppies go through a period of teething when the permanent teeth replace the puppy teeth. During this time, which culminates when he is four to six months old, your puppy will gnaw and chew at anything to soothe his sore and itching mouth. This is not 'biting.' As soon as he is no longer teething, he will no longer sink his needle-sharp teeth into your flesh. Don't waste your breath 'teaching' him not to bite. As I said, he isn't really biting at all; he is teething, and it will stop automatically – I absolutely guarantee it. Instead of wasting your time and compromising your relationship, simply spare your hands as much as possible by supplying other things for him to chew. A toy or a piece of cloth between your hand and his mouth is a perfect solution. For the rest, scratched and scarred hands are a sign that you have a teething puppy. Wear them with pride.

Bedtime
Puppies and kittens become overwhelmed and tired. Never disturb a sleeping puppy or kitten, and don't allow others to do so: children and guests will just have to wait for his batteries to recharge. When the sun sets on your first day together, remember that your puppy has had a big day, is away from everything he knows, and has probably never been completely alone. Ever. Until this point, he has spent every night of his life in a big, cosy, warm, living, breathing pile with his mother and siblings.

Together …
If you have already decided that, for the years

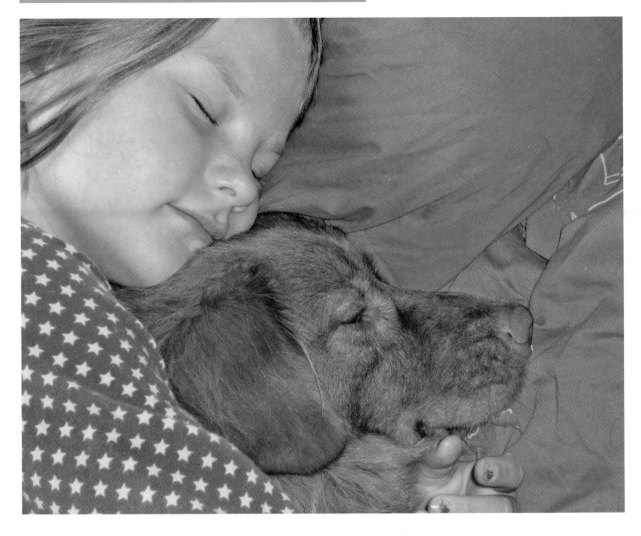

to come, your dog is welcome to sleep with you, either in your bed or in his own bed next to yours (preferably right next to yours, so you can spend the first few nights sleeping with one hand in his basket), the first night shouldn't be an issue at all. He will simply snuggle up with his new family, and you will have the added advantage, while he is still not house-trained, that you will likely notice the instant he wakes, and starts to move around during the night, allowing you to sweep him up and nip out for a pee break. If you can supervise him day and night to ensure that accidents don't happen, it is possible to have him fully house-trained within days.

… or alone

If, on the other hand, it is important to you to keep him out of your bed – maybe even out of your bedroom altogether – I suggest that you prepare to spend the first few nights sleeping beside him in his new bed. A mattress on the floor next to his bed for the first week allows him time to settle and feel safe in his new home, and it will generally mean that he will be happy by himself in his (now) familiar bed when you decide to move back to yours.

On one of your visits to the breeder, it's a good idea to leave a blanket, and ask that it go into the puppy pen for a few days before you arrive to pick up your puppy. This will give

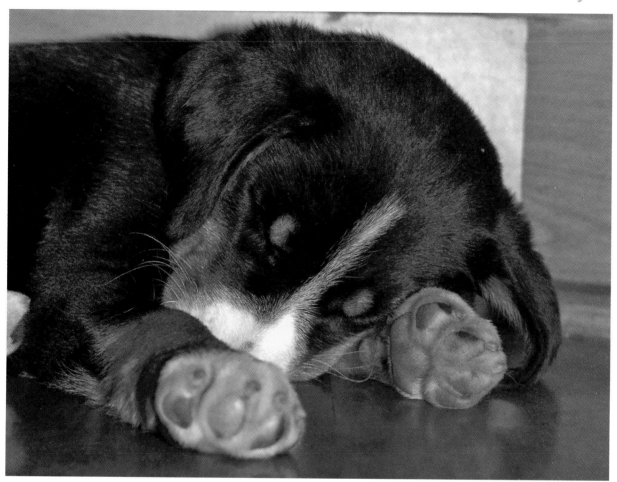

him a sense of home to snuggle up to during his first few nights in an alien environment, especially if he is shocked and upset at being left alone at night. A diffuser of calming pheromones (see page 214) in the room where he is to sleep can also help him feel relaxed and settled.

Finally, you may wish to say goodnight with a few drops of Dr Bach's Rescue Remedy on a treat at bedtime. If he is crying, you can try giving a dose of the homeopathic remedy Ignatia 200C or 1M, as this often helps a case of acute homesickness. You can read more about Bach flower remedies (see page 110) and homeopathy (see page 117) in the second part of this book.

If your puppy has to sleep alone from the outset, it may be a good idea to set your alarm to wake you halfway through the night so that you can take him out for a pee. Don't interact too much during these night-time toilet trips: they are just that; not a time for cuddling or playing games. Don't wait until his cries wake you up to take him out.

Dinnertime

It is very common for puppies to have diarrhoea during the first week in their new home. Make sure to get a supply of his usual food when you pick him up so that he doesn't have to cope with a change of diet on top of everything else. If you would like your puppy to eat a different diet than the food the breeder gave him, simply make a gradual change by replacing this with increasing amounts of your chosen food, starting a few weeks after he has settled into your home. Switching him to a raw diet, however, is generally best done in one go (see the chapter on diet (see page 34).

Puppies have small stomachs and thrive on eating little and often. A formula that works for most is to start him on three to four daily meals; reduce to two when he is at least six months old, and finally to one or two meals per day when he is fully grown. Remove any leftovers when he leaves the bowl or after half an hour if he likes to revisit his food for a while. He is less likely to grow up to be a picky eater if he learns from an early age to anticipate mealtimes with happy excitement.

Many dogs develop some degree of protective attitude around their food bowl and may growl if you get too close (food guarding). You can prevent this by simply making a point from the start of disturbing him regularly while he eats. Move his bowl around a bit while you add an extra delicious treat (such as a piece of meat) to his meal. In this way, he will, in no time at all, learn that being disturbed while he eats is no threat at all, but actually a very nice thing. If you have more than one dog, it is probably best to feed them separately. Even if they show no aggression toward each other at mealtimes, and are not interested in stealing each other's food, competition may cause them to overeat or gulp down their food.

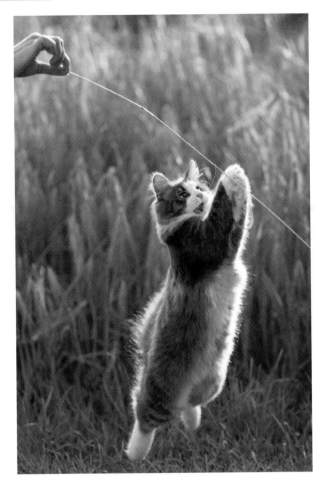

THE NEW KITTEN

Hello kitty!

I suspect that it isn't necessarily as stressful as one might imagine for a kitten to leave his mother and move to a new home. Cats are not social animals by nature, and your kitten may well be ready to go it alone. Even though cats tend to be solitary beings, this doesn't mean, of course, that they can't form strong bonds, or be sociable and loving toward one another, or that they don't enjoy the company of humans. Some cat lovers will point out that cats are, in fact, highly social animals, with evolved social structures that we are prone to overlook. Suffice to say that many cats appear to be very happy on their own, and are generally not dependent on social interaction in the same way as are dogs.

Calming pheromones (see page 214) and Dr Bach's Rescue Remedy (see page 111) can ease the transition if your kitten seems stressed or scared, perhaps because of the car ride home.

I recommend that you keep your kitten confined indoors initially. Even if he is eventually to have outdoor access, let him settle in and get his bearings before you let him out. If he bolts on his first outing because he is startled by another cat, a car or a low-flying jet, you want him to know his new home so that he runs back inside to seek refuge, instead of feeling lost in unknown surroundings and taking off in a blind panic. There are more reasons for keeping your kitten confined indoors for the first several months, and these are discussed in the chapter on neutering on page 89. Also see the chapters on vaccination and diet for information on how to look after your kitten's health.

Another one joins the clowder

Kittens tend to settle into new surroundings without problems. When problems do arise, it is usually because there are already cats living in the household. A group of cats is sometimes referred to as a clowder (in case you were wondering). Whatever you call it, if you already share your home with one or more cats and decide to introduce a new kitten, be aware that this may constitute a conflict of interests.

People like to keep several cats together, whereas they tend to be solitary by nature, so keeping several cats in close proximity may be a cause of stress. In most cases, two or more cats will coexist happily, but the introduction of a new kitten will, at least temporarily, upset the balance, and may induce a stress reaction in the others, even when they don't seem to be reacting strongly to the newcomer. Make sure that all of the cats are able to get away from each other, find privacy, and avoid stressful encounters. There are several steps you can take in an attempt to ensure a smooth transition. Read more about cats and stress on pages 165 and 207, about stress-reducing supplements on page 210, and about Bach flower remedies and homeopathy in the second part of this book.

Recognising cat stress

The introduction of a new cat will invariably change the dynamic in the group, which may cause stress in one or more of the cats. When cats suffer from stress, very often the only signs are physical in the form of either urinary symptoms (peeing outside the litter tray or even overt cystitis), or skin symptoms (over-grooming to the point of creating bald spots or ulcers). If you see any of these symptoms, be aware that they are common expressions of stress in cats. You can read more about solving these issues in the sections on urinary problems and skin disease in the third part of this book.

PUPPY AND KITTEN HEALTH

Just like human babies, puppies and kittens have immature immune systems that are still acclimatising and learning about the world. This will invariably lead to innocuous infections such as conjunctivitis, diarrhoea and the odd rash in young individuals of any species. Their immune systems are further challenged by the fact that puppies and kittens are moved to an entirely new environment and by the unavoidable physical and psychological stress caused by such an upheaval.

Poor timing

In many countries, it is, unfortunately, customary to vaccinate puppies and kittens immediately prior to rehoming. While it is understandable that breeder and buyer alike see it as a sign of responsible breeding practice that the youngsters receive their first vaccine before they are sent out into the world, it is often actually very poor timing.

We know that there is a period of unspecific suppression of the immune system from day three to day ten following vaccination. You could say that the immune system, faced with several deadly diseases, momentarily needs to focus on this challenge, and therefore takes its eye off the ball in terms of its day-to-day job of maintaining health. This is not a side effect of vaccination but merely a consequence of the vaccine stimulating the immune system, as it is supposed to do.

This means, however, that someone who has just received a vaccine is, for a period of ten days or so, less protected than they were before, so choosing this exact time to uproot a kitten or puppy and introduce him into a completely new environment is somewhat unfortunate timing. The first week in a new home is probably the one week in their life when they most need a well-functioning and strong immune system. In the chapter on vaccination (see page 51), I discuss ways to avoid this unfortunate situation.

The homeopathic remedy Thuja 200C is always indicated as immune support when someone is vaccinated (see page 49 on using Thuja in this context). The herb echinacea is also a great supplement for supporting the immune system during this vulnerable time. Give a few drops of echinacea herbal tincture on a treat two to three times daily. If your puppy or kitten's digestion is affected, adding a probiotic (beneficial gut bacteria) to his diet for a few weeks is also a good idea.

Diarrhoea

There are many reasons why newly-rehomed puppies and kittens often suffer from diarrhoea: immune suppression following vaccination, diet change from milk to solids, possible introduction of new foods and treats when they move to a new home, combined with all the physical and psychological stressors of being completely uprooted and moved to a new environment. All of these factors and more combine to make this a sensitive and vulnerable period.

If your puppy gets diarrhoea, remove any dry food and change instead to an easily digestible, low-fat diet (rice or mashed potatoes with chicken being the classic), which should be fed frequently and in small amounts. 'Little and often' is a good rule to bear in mind,

as a small amount every couple of hours is generally tolerated much better than large meals. Make sure he drinks, and do give him a probiotic supplement. In a case of diarrhoea without vomiting, the probiotic products that come in a tube are ideal. These are widely available from veterinary clinics and pet shops, and are good to keep on hand, just in case.

Homeopathic treatment can also provide invaluable support for digestion during this transition period. You can read about homeopathic treatment and how to use it in the second part of this book, but, if your puppy gets diarrhoea during the first few days, I suggest that you try giving him the homeopathic remedy Capsicum 30C. Dr Bach's Rescue Remedy is also worth trying as it has a specific effect on symptoms caused by acute stress. If the diarrhoea is watery and your puppy is also vomiting, the homeopathic remedy Arsenicum album may fit the picture. You can read more about acute diarrhoea on page 168.

If the stools contain blood or mucus, if the diarrhoea continues for more than a couple of days, or if at any point your puppy or kitten becomes weak or dehydrated, see the vet immediately. In most cases of puppy diarrhoea, however, this isn't necessary.

THE FIRST VISIT TO THE VET

A word of warning: don't fall for the 'health club,' 'health plan' or other loyalty schemes that many veterinary clinics offer. These are invariably based on giving a superfluous number of vaccines and parasite treatments: avoid them as you would avoid anyone who still refers to the 'annual vaccination' (there is no such thing!). Choose informed, bespoke veterinary advice instead of schemes pushing treatments that your animals don't need. They will be healthier, and you will end up giving fewer treatments (thus probably even saving money).

In my hometown, a local veterinary hospital advertises its scheme via a campaign posted on local buses. Their advert states that 'every fourth vaccine is free,' but given that few dogs need four vaccines in their lifetime, more than once this has given me cause to practice a few breathing exercises when stuck in traffic.

The puppy visit

In many cases, your puppy will already be microchipped, and have received his first vaccination when you pick him up from the breeder. You may wish to take him to the vet within a few days anyway, just to have him checked over, introduce puppy to vet and vet to puppy, and ask the vet's advice on all the questions that come with getting to know your new puppy.

Alternatively, you may decide to wait three to four weeks, until it is time for a vaccination, before you take your puppy on his first trip to the vet's. You may also have decided to postpone the first vaccination until your pup has settled into his new environment, or indeed you may rely on titre testing to determine the optimal timing of his puppy vaccination. In any case, you will be seeing your vet within a month of your puppy's arrival. Microchip and health insurance are probably already taken care of at this time; if not, be sure to ask your vet about these. This is also the time to get advice about worming, and to bring up any other questions or concerns that may have arisen during your first days or weeks together (a list may help you remember your questions). If you have not already signed up for puppy classes, your vet probably knows who to recommend in your area, so put that on the list, too.

There is a lot to say about vaccination, so please read the chapter beginning on page 42 before taking your puppy to the vet for the first time. All puppies should be vaccinated against distemper, parvovirus and hepatitis. If you live in an area where rabies is prevalent

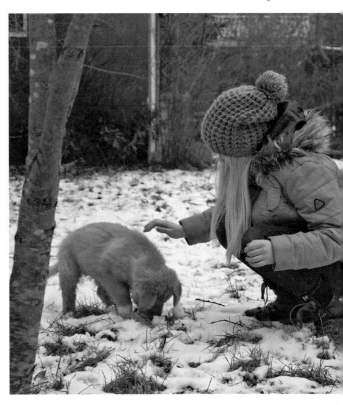

in the wild animal population, your puppy may need a rabies vaccine, too. In Australia, New Zealand, the UK, and most other European countries, vaccination against rabies is not relevant unless you are planning to travel with your puppy. If your travel plans are vague or you are not leaving for a few months, postpone the rabies vaccine until a month before travel. In any case, separate it from the other puppy vaccines by at least two to three weeks (preferably much longer) if at all possible. It is worth an extra trip to the vet's to space out the vaccines in order not to over-burden your animal's immune system. Don't forget to give the homeopathic remedy Thuja around the time of vaccination. See more about this on page 49 and where to get your Thuja on page 216.

Unvaccinated puppies should never be isolated. If you would like to join a puppy class but find that its regulations won't allow your puppy to join until he has had his puppy shot(s) (one or more puppy vaccines may be needed, depending on timing and use of titre testing; see page 51), and if they won't listen to reason, simply find another class. Fortunately, vaccination policy has been updated in many places, but you will still find the occasional misinformed dog trainer. Don't let that force your hand. The puppy most at risk is actually the newly-vaccinated one. If anyone is to skip training, it should be the puppy who was vaccinated within the past ten days. Even then, I tend to think that socialisation comes first, so, provided he is not feeling under the weather, I would let him out to play.

The kitten visit

Apart from the general points made above, let me mention here the vaccines that your kitten will need at some point, depending on his lifestyle. Please also read the relevant chapters on vaccination, diet and neutering.

If your kitten has outdoor access from the start, he should be vaccinated as soon as possible against cat flu and panleukopenia (also called cat parvovirus). You should also ensure that he (or she) is neutered before reaching sexual maturity, which usually happens at around the age of five to six months. If your kitten is to lead an indoor life, it is your choice whether or not to vaccinate, and you can usually wait longer before neutering. Even if he is to be an indoor cat, however, it is a good idea to at least give the panleukopenia vaccine and to let him have a microchip or ear tattoo. This could save his life if the day comes when he escapes through an open window. All kittens, regardless of lifestyle, need worming treatments.

Diet

Factory food, home cooked or raw?

What shall I feed my dog? Which is the best brand of cat food? These are questions I get asked a lot. The only possible answer to such questions is: 'That all depends on the animal.' Individual consideration is always crucial, so it must be the case that no diet is ideal for everyone.

Sick animals may need special dietary considerations: see the sections on kidney disease and gastro-intestinal disease in the third part of this book for further discussion of the role of diet in these conditions. This chapter deals only with the care of healthy adult animals – but still, no diet fits all.

If you do a little research on diet for dogs or cats, one problem you'll almost certainly encounter is that there is next to no available research or published information that isn't produced by someone with an idea or product to sell. Independent expert nutritional advice is very hard to come by. Formation of the Raw Feeding Veterinary Society (RFVS) is a step toward correcting this, with vets from all over the world working together to collect and distribute independent advice on raw feeding.

In my opinion, looking at the anatomy of the digestive tract of a dog or cat, and considering the diet of their wild ancestors, is the most logical approach to understanding their ideal diet. So, as a sound starting point, let's look at what makes a diet appropriate to each species.

FEEDING A FELINE – THE MEAT EATER WHO FORGETS TO DRINK

Cats need meat

Cats are obligate carnivores, which means that, whatever form it comes in, they need meat. As strict carnivores, cats rely on nutrients in animal tissue to meet their specific and unique nutritional requirements. There are certain amino acids, most famously taurine, that cats cannot synthesize, and which must therefore be present in their diet. This means that feeding a vegetarian diet to a cat is as unnatural as serving up steak to a horse.

Cats can't even live on standard dog food, as it simply doesn't contain enough meat. They thrive, however, on a diet consisting exclusively of meat. Unfortunately, this isn't what most cats are being offered.

Not thirsty

The ancestors of our domestic cat evolved in arid, desert-like landscapes. As a result, cats are to this day equipped with extremely efficient kidneys, able to preserve water by concentrating their urine much more than do the kidneys of humans or dogs. Therefore, by their nature, they are not really interested in drinking, and are simply designed to get all of the fluid they need from their fresh prey, rather than having to search out a watering hole (or

indeed, a water bowl). Yes, if you feed your cat dry food, he will drink, but, because of his naturally low thirst drive, he still won't drink enough.

Studies have measured the water intake of cats fed a diet of tinned cat food (water content 75%: roughly the same as in fresh prey), and found that, when the diet is changed to dry food, the cats certainly do drink more, but are able to increase their water intake only enough to make up about half the difference.

To put it bluntly, a cat on a dry diet (as most are) is chronically dehydrated: he simply cannot drink enough to keep up.

What's the harm?

Please hold on to these two important facts about cats –

* They have evolved to get fluid from their food rather than through drinking
* They are by nature strict meat-eaters

Most cats are fed factory-made cat food in either a wet form, bought in tins or pouches, or in dry form as kibble. *Neither fulfils the above two basic requirements.* I am convinced that cats suffer much more than dogs or other animal species from health problems as a direct consequence of a species-inappropriate diet.

Problem number one: cats and drinking

Fresh prey, such as a bird or mouse, consists of about 75% liquid: roughly the same as tinned cat food (and, yes, that is an expensive way to buy water, but that is for another day). Dry, pelleted, factory-produced cat food (kibble) contains only around 10% liquid – that's a lot of extra water requirement to make up for someone who doesn't easily feel thirst. It is clear, then, that wet cat food, from the point of view of maintaining a healthy fluid balance, is far superior to dry food.

Does it really matter so much if cats drink too little?

The urinary system is the main problem area for cats, and cystitis and urinary stones are serious and common ailments. And isn't the kidney the organ that invariably fails in elderly cats? Dogs, humans and horses don't have anywhere near the same incidence of kidney disease as do cats. A diet high in moisture increases a cat's total water intake to a degree that cannot be achieved by feeding a dry diet and leaving fresh water available. If we leave it up to the cat, he simply won't drink enough.

You have to wonder, who thought it would be a good idea to feed cats dehydrated food? Now that we know the trouble it causes, let's stop. A higher daily water intake results in increased urine volume and dilution, which has been shown to reduce the risk of urinary disease in cats. In short, if you want to prevent bladder and kidney disease, don't feed your cat dry food. (See also the chapter on diseases of the urinary system, page 178). A constant state of dehydration may well explain why the urinary system is such a problem area for cats. There are other explanations for this (see the chapter on vaccination, page 46), but there can be no doubt that the dry food that most of us feed to our cats has a lot to answer for in terms of potential long-term health complications.

Problem number two: cats and carbohydrates

Processed cat food, whether dry or wet, generally contains far too much carbohydrate, and the unique way that cats break down, digest and utilise their food is simply not designed for carbohydrates. Adult cats require two to three times more protein in their diet than do adult dogs. Good-quality animal protein is, unfortunately, expensive, so you can safely assume that the cheaper the cat food, the higher the content of carbohydrate (wheat, potato, soy, corn), and the lower the content of good-quality meat.

The unique nutritional needs of cats as true carnivores mean that their natural requirement is a high-protein, moderate-fat, low-carbohydrate diet. This is, if you like, the paleo diet for cats: a nutritional approach that considers genetics. This is what their gastrointestinal tract is designed to process. When we feed them a diet high in carbohydrate and relatively low in animal protein, we inadvertently create a multitude of problems. Widespread inappropriate (ie high-carbohydrate) feeding of cats may contribute to obesity, diabetes, liver disease, and inflammatory bowel disease.

In contrast to dogs, most cats diagnosed with diabetes suffer from type 2 (insulin-resistant) diabetes. Some diabetic cats are cured simply by being put on a meat-only diet, but note that this is absolutely NOT something to experiment with at home if your cat is already receiving insulin, or has just been diagnosed with diabetes, but it does illustrate how important it is to consider diet when cats fall ill. Always involve your vet, and if your vet is not open to a discussion – for instance about switching a diabetic cat to a raw-food diet – see the chapter on page 37.

But my cat is doing fine!

We probably all know cats who are fed exclusively on own-brand supermarket dry cat food, and seem to be doing absolutely fine. How can that be? Firstly, not all cats on this less-than-ideal diet will develop urinary disease, colitis or diabetes, though far too many will develop these and other lifestyle health problems. People get away with junk food diets, too. Secondly, thriving – being in optimal health – is not the same as surviving without visible signs of malnourishment or disease. You can buy vegan cat food if you wish, although, in my opinion, you should get a pet with longer ears if you feel that meat-based pet food is not ethically defensible (an argument I do have a lot of sympathy for, though this doesn't change the fact that cats are carnivores, regardless of how we may feel about it). Thirdly, everyone with a problem was doing great until suddenly they weren't. There is a long period where health is compromised before symptoms appear and a disease is diagnosed. For some, it never happens, but the fact that some cope with a substandard diet shouldn't be used as an argument to support it.

So, how do we go about giving cats a species-appropriate diet?

Nobody tells a cat what to do
First of all, it doesn't matter what I decide to feed my cat if the cat is not on board with this. You can't tell a cat what to do. Cats are creatures of habit, and if a cat has not been eating a varied diet from a young age, getting him to try something new can pose a real challenge. Never get into a battle over this. A tough, you-will-eat-it-when-you-get-hungry-enough approach won't work, and not eating, even for a few days, can make a cat very ill. You simply cannot be more stubborn than your cat.

What you can be is more patient, which is a lot easier if you know what to expect. See page 34 for tips on transitioning your cat onto a new diet.

A DOG'S DINNER — ABLE TO ADAPT BUT STILL A CARNIVORE AT HEART

Dogs are facultative carnivores, which means that their digestive system is that of a carnivore, and they thrive on a meat-based diet, but are also able to synthesize protein from other energy sources, and can therefore survive without meat. That is not to say that this is ideal, or that any dog would ever *choose* to become vegetarian. Dogs have the teeth and the short digestive tract of a meat-eater.

I have often noticed that, when I speak

to a processed-food company rep who has come to the veterinary clinic to promote their brand of kibble, or to a petshop owner selling raw foods, they can sound quite similar in their conviction that, without this particular food, doggie doom is inevitable. I take a somewhat more relaxed position. It is actually quite hard to feed a dog a diet so hopeless that the dog will suffer and become visibly malnourished. Dogs (at least adult dogs) are very forgiving in this way, and able to live on a broad spectrum of diets. In all my years as a vet, I remember seeing only one instance of a dog who was clearly suffering from malnutrition: this dog was fed a vegan diet consisting only of raw whole vegetables and, as a consequence, was severely underweight and suffering from heart disease.

My point is that dogs may be more forgiving than cats when it comes to diet, but surely it goes for any species that eating a diet that covers basic nutritional needs and avoids overt illness from malnourishment is one thing, whilst eating an ideal diet that leaves an animal thriving and in optimal health is quite another – just as humans may survive on junk food, but will probably live better on a varied, organic diet of unprocessed and wholesome foods.

THE OPTIONS

So, what are the options when it comes to feeding dogs and cats?

There are, simply put, three different ways you can feed your dog or cat: processed factory food, homemade food, and raw food.

What follows is a look at the pros and cons of each approach, and tips to improve the diet that works best for you.

• PROCESSED FACTORY FOOD

Certainly easier ...
Processed food comes in wet form in tins or

pouches and in dry form as pellets (kibble), and has to be the easiest way to feed your pet. The shelf life is long, and in a busy household, convenience is certainly a valid factor when making lifestyle choices. Factory pet food, whether wet or dry, requires no preparation, and is easily stored at room temperature (if dry) and in a fridge once opened (if wet), making it the most suitable diet for travelling, for those with limited time or space, and those who don't wish to handle meat. Just open the tin or reach into the bag and feed.

... but not inherently better

The pet-food industry has achieved a remarkable feat: on some level, convincing us that preparing pet food is rocket science, and far beyond the common sense allocated to mere mortals. There is a very widespread belief that laboratory scientists in white coats must know best, and that they have developed a product that is far superior to the simple food to which the rest of us have access.

The truth, if we pause to think about it, is that this is an industry that produces a product for profit. There is nothing wrong with that, but let's not be brainwashed into thinking that this product is somehow superior to real food. There are artificial additives in most dry foods to prevent the fats turning rancid, and to ensure a shelf life of many months, and some of these additives are under suspicion of having potentially serious side effects. The main ingredients used in the pet food industry are often selected based on what was cheap on the world market at the time of manufacture, and the legal requirements are concerned with minimum dietary requirements only. Convenience pet food is simple and easy, and it can be a perfectly adequate choice, but in absolutely no way is it *better*.

Don't make this choice because you think anything else is too complicated. The nutritional value of processed foods is not superior in any way. Just pause for a moment

to consider how crazy it is that we are led to believe that leftover, fresh, prime-quality meat from our dinner plates should be thrown away rather than fed to the dog. Do you think that a product using whatever animal tissue (probably ending up in pet food in the first place because it was deemed unfit for human consumption), which has been highly processed to the point where the original ingredients are unrecognisable, and then stored in a bag for months and months, is somehow a healthier choice for our dogs and cats than human-grade fresh meat?

When I put it that way, probably not. Yet I often hear people proudly state that, at *their* house, all leftovers go straight in the bin because dogs should, of course, have only dog food. This idea is the result of marketing so refined that it almost amounts to brainwashing.

We have all been there. Contrary to common belief, most vets don't recommend certain brands of dog or cat food just because they can make a profit selling it to you: more often than not, they genuinely believe in the superiority of the product. Nutrition as taught at vet school often directly involves the pet food companies, yet human nutritionists tell *us* to eat a varied, unprocessed, and preferably organic diet. If it were possible to put together a freeze-dried pellet that covered all of our nutritional requirements in a way that was markedly superior to fresh produce, I am sure we would all be advised to eat that. As it is, unless you are climbing mountains or flying to the moon, chances are you are not eating a highly processed pellet put together by experts a year ago. Ready-made complete pet food in either wet or dry form is an easy and convenient way to feed your dog or cat, and it is often perfectly adequate. It is not, however, in any way nutritionally preferable to *real* food.

You (sometimes) get what you pay for ...

Processed food varies greatly in quality. I have

seen more than one example of consumer tests analysing pet foods, and concluding that they all live up to legal requirements, and so we, the consumer, are advised to buy the cheapest, the clear implication being that if we buy anything but the cheapest brand we are being conned. The reason for this ill-founded advice is that these consumer tests assess the foods against minimal requirements, meaning that all they are really saying is that none of the foods will lead to disease from malnourishment. Needless to say, this does not mean they are all of equal quality.

Read the label ...

Do read ingredient lists. By law, the ingredients have to be listed in descending order by weight. A good starting point, therefore, is to go for a brand that lists meat first. Even then there are some pitfalls. Fresh meat is 75% water, so once the product has been dried, meat may no longer be the main ingredient. Also, consider that a label listing, for instance, 'chicken, maize, wheat, rice, soy' sounds like a great product containing meat as its main ingredient, but actually may well consist of 21% chicken, 20% maize, 20% wheat, 20% rice and 19% soy, making it nearly 80% carbohydrate. 'Grain-free' is another promising label that could turn out to describe a product consisting primarily of potato. Although the quality of the meat used is almost impossible to ascertain, a good guide to identifying a superior product is to look for those with the highest meat content and the shortest list of ingredients. These will invariably be the most expensive brands. You do get what you pay for, and meat is what you are after. Everything else is just filler.

... and don't be seduced

The benefits claimed are many and fanciful, and reading pet food labels can be entertaining or exasperating, depending on your mood. Ingredients that no dog or cat would ever think appetising increasingly find their way into upmarket pet foods. Herbs, exotic fruits and berries are, somewhat randomly, added for that wholesome feeling that is likely to appeal to the human buying the product. There can be no doubt that the orange added to the duck variety is included to entice the person buying the food, not the animal eating it. Likewise, blueberries are no doubt healthy and look good on the label, but I am not sure that being heated, smashed, dried and then stored for a year leaves much goodness to be absorbed.

These days, you can buy specific foods for different ages, breeds, health conditions ... I wouldn't be surprised to learn that someone had launched a new dry food for each day of the week. Imagine, just for fun, supermarket shelves displaying different pasta sauces for different human age groups, genders or body types ('this sauce is specifically designed for short men over 40 with a tendency to heart and knee problems').

I have very little faith that the supplements added to the mix have any effect at all after the product has been processed and subsequently stored at room temperature for many months. The label says these have been added, and this is no doubt true. If your dog or cat need oils, herbs or other supplements, I strongly recommend that you add them yourself. This way, you can control the amount as well as ensure that the supplements you choose are appropriate, fresh, and of the highest quality.

• HOMEMADE FOOD

Dogs have existed on human scraps for thousands of years, and it is still perfectly fine to feed your dogs and cats as members of the family. I absolutely disagree with the common mantra that 'pets should not eat human food.' Don't feed them junk, of course, and be aware of the few foods that are potentially toxic to animals (listed in the table below).

Cats are meat-eaters and should be fed meat, either raw or cooked. Some cats have a surprising liking for certain fruits or vegetables, which is fine, but the main diet must be meat. Dogs, on the other hand, can eat whatever is being served in terms of rice, potatoes, pasta, bread, salads and vegetables, provided you remember that at least half of their daily diet should be meat. Sometimes, a nice-sounding staple diet of 'chicken and rice' actually turns out to mean rice with a bit of chicken added for flavour – this is not a suitable diet. It's a good rule of thumb that at least half of the dog bowl by bulk should be taken up by meat.

It is still my experience that there are dog owners who throw prime steak into the bin because they believe that dogs must not have leftovers, and should eat only 'dog food,' and I would very much like to correct this misunderstanding. There can be no doubt that the nutritional value of the meat and vegetables from our dinner tables far exceeds that of the ingredients that go into dog food. Don't feed the fatty rind of meat (this can be a burden for the pancreas), and don't feed overly-spicy foods. Apart from that, just be aware of the few human foods and additives that are potentially toxic to dogs and cats, remember to provide enough meat, and trust that feeding your dog is a matter of common sense, just like feeding yourself and the rest of your family.

Remember ...

If you are feeding a varied homecooked diet, remember this rule of thumb: At least half of your dog's meal should consist of meat. There is no upper limit. For an adult, healthy dog, feeding only meat is perfectly fine.

RAW FOOD

A raw meat diet is often referred to as BARF, which originally stood for 'bones and raw food,' but seems to have been reinvented as 'biologically appropriate raw food,' and refers to the increasingly common practice of feeding raw meat, sometimes as a 100% raw meat diet; sometimes supplemented with vegetables.

This movement, as I am almost tempted to call it, was started by the Australian veterinary surgeon Ian Billinghurst, whose book *Give your dog a bone*, published in 1993, argued that dogs should be fed meat, preferably raw, meaty bones. Since then, a whole industry has grown up around selling ready-to-feed frozen meat for dogs and cats.

To my mind, a raw food diet has to be the most natural approach to feeding cats and dogs, carnivorous species that they are: it just makes good sense to provide what dogs and cats have been eating for thousands and thousands of years. It is hard to argue against the fact that, as their digestive systems were clearly developed to eat raw meat, this is the most species-appropriate diet we can offer them. A Chihuahua may no longer look like a wolf on the outside, but he is still a carnivore on the inside. Even if evolving alongside humans may have enabled dogs to eat more carbohydrate, uncooked meat is still the

Never let your dog or cat have ...

- onion, spring onion, leek or garlic
- grapes or raisins
- chocolate or cocoa
- nuts, especially macadamia nuts
- avocado
- anything containing the sweetener xylitol

Contact your vet immediately if your animal has eaten any of the above foods. Don't wait for symptoms to show

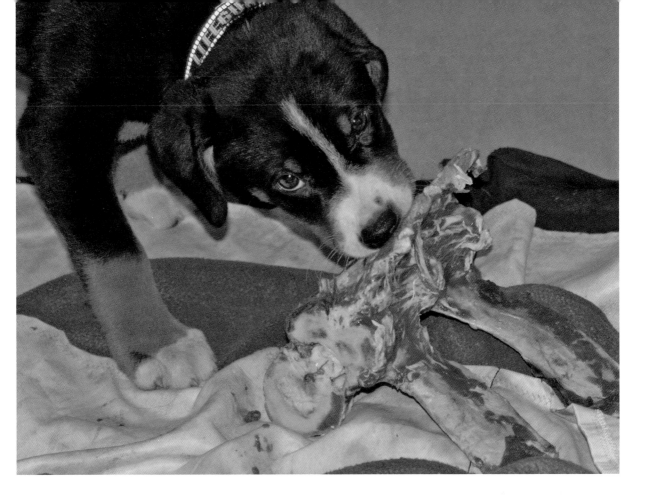

original dog food, and has been so since early dog.

In comparison, processed kibble and tinned, cooked dog food has been around for less than a century.

But what about the hassle ...

Feeding raw meat doesn't have to be a bloodbath; nor do you have to be a hunter, a butcher, or even the slightest bit handy with a meat cleaver. Of course, you may be able to liaise with a local farmer or butcher, but everything you need is available at your local supermarket's meat counter. Easier still, a multitude of companies now supply meal-sized packages of raw frozen meat – some even deliver straight to your freezer.

Unless you live close to a veterinary clinic or pet shop that sells frozen meat, or are happy to shop for meat at the supermarket several times a week, suitable freezer space is probably the biggest hurdle to raw feeding. Once you have a freezer full of meat, picking out a bag of food to defrost for tomorrow as you put down the bowl of today's raw meat is really as quick and easy as reaching into a bag of factory-made, processed petfood. No preparation involved at all.

... and the mess

If you feed ground raw meat (available with or without ground bone), you simply shake out the required amount from the bag into the bowl for defrosting, and there will be no mess involved at all. Of course, you may like to feed raw meaty bones (see page 32 regarding cooked/uncooked bones), which requires some space (or at least a sheet on the floor) to limit the mess. Some dogs, like my own, would prefer to take the bones off somewhere to gnaw in peace, or to bury for later enjoyment. A half-eaten raw chicken leg under your pillow helps you remember not to leave doors open during feeding time.

We are so used to giving our pets processed meals that can be inhaled straight from the bowl in a few minutes, that we forget the occupational value and deep satisfaction a dog gets from lying down for half-an-hour or more to thoroughly chew a large, meaty bone. In a garden or a yard, on a balcony or with a sheet on the floor – whatever your housing situation, occasional bone-chewing is possible in most circumstances, and will be greatly appreciated by your dog.

... and the risks

The frowning vet

Some vets strongly support BARF feeding, and many veterinary clinics even supply the meat. Others are hellbent against it. If your vet is very set against raw feeding, and it is your chosen approach, I suggest you find another vet. You need to be able to be honest, and it isn't helpful or constructive to have the same discussion every time you visit, or indeed, to have a vet who blames any illness on the raw feeding (believe me, it happens!), or who will refuse to feed your dog's usual food if he is ever hospitalised. Find a vet who shares your approach. See page 37 for the importance of finding the right vet for you.

The Raw Feeding Veterinary Society (RFVS) is a good starting point for finding a vet who supports your choice of diet.

The germs

Life is full of risks, but, in my experience, there is no particular risk involved in raw feeding.

Naturally, you will need to observe usual hygiene around raw meat: don't spill blood on the salad in your fridge; don't let your toddler use the dog's dinner as finger paint, and do wash up the feeding bowl in hot, soapy water. If you are used to handling and cooking meat,

this won't be news to you, and there is no need for extra precautions.

From time to time, the press will feature headlines proclaiming that raw meat has been found to contain bacteria (well, yes) or that a dog eating raw meat is a health risk, as he may spread disease by licking a baby's face. I'm sorry, but there is only one reasonable response to these scare-mongering stories: yes, of course raw meat will contain bacteria such as salmonella (hence the precautions above), but the carnivore's stomach acid, digestive enzymes, and short intestinal passage means that these won't make your dog ill, and, if you handle the meat like any raw meat should be handled, it won't make you ill either.

If dogs couldn't digest raw meat, there would be no dogs in the world (and what a sad state of affairs that would be). As for the dog eating raw meat and then licking your baby's face, I really don't see the problem when you compare that to the kibble-fed dog who just gnawed on a dead bird in the garden, sniffed another dog's bum, or maybe just snaffled a morsel of tasty excrement on the morning walk ...?

Bone of contention

Cooked bone will splinter into sharp fragments, and most vets have seen the damage that can be done to a dog's intestines by the shards of bone that were once the Sunday roast chicken. This is the reason why many people, including many vets, turn pale at the mention of feeding bone in any form. It is, however, crucial to differentiate between raw and cooked bone.

Never feed cooked bones. Raw bones are a totally different story, however, as they are digestible, and generally don't cause any problem at all. It is common sense to supervise your dog when he is eating bones. If he is of an excitable disposition and tends to gobble everything without chewing, you can help him learn to chew, rather than swallow whole, by initially feeding only large bones, or by holding the end of the bone. Of course, it is possible for a dog to choke on a piece of bone, just as he can choke on a chew or a toy, but with common sense this is very rarely a problem. If the thought of raw bones doesn't appeal to you, perhaps due to the mess on the kitchen floor, you can buy BARF meat with ground-up bone added. This does, however, mean that your dog misses out on most of the benefit to gums and teeth that come from regular bone-gnawing.

Feeding bones

Cooked bones and raw bones are two completely different things. Whereas meat can be fed cooked or raw, cooked bones should be avoided, as these can splinter and cause serious internal damage. Raw bones are generally digested well, and don't tend to cause problems.

... and the benefits

For everyone

Everyone benefits from good nutrition, and a change to BARF often makes a dramatic difference in the symptoms of dogs and cats suffering from obesity, or from digestive issues such as recurrent vomiting or diarrhoea. In my experience, however, the claims of an alleged effect on animals suffering from skin allergies are often somewhat exaggerated. Some are certainly helped but many are not, because most allergic dogs and cats are not primarily allergic to food (see page 159 on allergies).

Young or old, sick or healthy, most will feel the general health benefits from a healthy diet. Of course, some dogs don't thrive on a raw meat diet, and I cannot emphasise enough the importance of observing each particular animal rather than being guided by a pre-conceived notion about what is 'best.' We are all different, with individual preferences and needs, and so are our dogs.

Meaningful occupation

Apart from the nutritional aspect, there are other benefits to feeding raw meaty bones. When you give your dog a bone, you also give him a chance to act on his instincts.

Chewing on a bone is a meaningful occupation for a dog. Imagine the life of a wild dog, spending most of his time hunting, then eating the prey, digesting the meal and going back to hunting. Compare that with our domestic pet dog, who is lkely to be fed meals that can be inhaled from a bowl in a few minutes. The daily walk may take up an hour. That leaves around 23 hours without meaningful occupation or stimulation. For many dogs, most of this time is even spent home alone. No surprise, then, when dogs develop destructive behaviour such as chewing on shoes or furniture, and an indoor cat over-eats his dry food out of boredom.

Raw sense

Raw meat should not be left out for hours, and I recommend that dry food that isn't eaten within half an hour should be removed as well. Raw meat in any form contains bacteria that can make you sick. Simple hygiene precautions, such as washing up the bowl after each meal, storing raw meat separately from other food, and washing your hands and utensils after handling raw meat should prevent any problems.

Natural dental hygiene

As a vet, I struggle to bring myself to advise against tooth brushing for dogs and cats, although, if pressed, I will admit that I have always found it a bit silly. We feed them mush or small pellets that even a toothless dog or cat could eat, and then lecture about the need for toothbrushing and artificial chews to deal with the problems we create. The teeth of a carnivore are made for tearing skin and flesh, chewing raw meat and crunching bone. Why not let them do just that?

Anal sacs

Anal sac problems are described in the last section of this book (see page 172). Blocked anal sacs often result from stools being too soft; a problem easily resolved by changing to a BARF diet. Most people find that their dogs poo much less often in this case, and that the stools are firm and dry in consistency, exactly as nature intended for optimal function of the anal glands.

MAKING THE CHANGE

If your animals are used to dry food and you decide to change their diet – either to wet processed food or to raw food – you may need to prepare for a period of transition. Most dogs enthusiastically welcome a change from kibble to real food, and there is no reason for it to be a gradual transition. Starve them for a day and then simply change to raw. There is plenty of advice out there on how best to do this whilst avoiding constipation or diarrhoea in the first weeks. See the list of references on page 217.

Sometimes, an elderly or ill dog with sensitive digestion may not be able to eat both processed dry food and raw food, and therefore may need to stick to a purely raw-meat diet. He may also need a more careful transition, perhaps initially relying on frequent meals of bone broth. Speak to an holistic vet; she can give you all the help you need.

Many cats, especially those mature enough to be set in their ways, will need some convincing. If you have gone to the trouble of reading up on the benefits of a BARF diet for your cat, you have bought the meat, you have served it up expectantly – and now your cat is not only refusing to eat, but giving you a decidedly evil look as well (much like the

reaction of a teenager used to burgers upon being offered an organic salad). The natural reaction is to give up and conclude that your cat won't eat raw meat.

Better to be prepared for this eventuality. It takes patience, creativity, and a sense of humour to beat your cat at this game. Never simply remove the old food, leaving him the choice between the new diet and starvation. More often than not, starve he will, and that can make a cat very ill, very quickly. The only road to a successful transition is gentle persuasion (I think the term is nudging, but we can call it manipulation if you like). Never, ever, try to force him.

The way to a cat's stomach

The first, and probably most important step, is the introduction of mealtimes. We want to generate a sense of excitement and anticipation about food. You may be there already, but if your cat is used to having free access to dry food around the clock, start by removing the bowl, and, without changing the diet, introducing mealtimes once or twice a day. Whatever food is left over after half an hour is removed until the next meal.

Don't worry if your cat is a bit confused for the first few days. If he eats less than a full ration for a week or two, that will only sharpen his focus and interest in mealtimes. As long as he eats something, he will be fine.

Stay with the familiar diet until mealtimes are an established routine. Once he comes running, excited by the prospect of a meal, offer a small amount of the new food and leave him with that for a little while. Hungry, and expecting food, he will at the very least show some interest, and sniff it before deciding it is not acceptable. Then you simply feed his meal as usual.

If you keep this up, after a period of sniffing and rejecting the unfamiliar food before eating his usual diet, he will start to lick it before rejecting it, moving gradually (and this can take months, so be patient) to tasting it.

If you have a greedy cat, you may get away with an even simpler approach by leaving a small piece of meat on a separate plate whenever you happen to be cooking meat. He can then sniff it and reject it, and you can throw it away and repeat the following day.

It's very easy to become discouraged and give up within a week if you invest too much in this project. You don't want to shop for lots of varieties of new food only to see them all rejected, and conclude that your cat won't eat them. Offer a tiny piece of meat whenever you are cooking it for yourself anyway, or, if you don't eat meat, you can freeze ice cube-sized bits to offer (and then most likely discard) on a daily basis.Sometimes, staying with one initial source of protein (eg rabbit or chicken) helps.

Some cats like to start with slightly cooked warm meat that gives off an appetising scent. Patience is the key. If you only give it a week and your cat doesn't happen to be Garfield, you will fail. It may take six months, but it won't demand much effort on your part, and your cat will be much healthier when you get there.

If your cat is not addicted to dry food, but is already happily eating tinned cat food, it is often possible to simply substitute increasing amounts with raw minced meat. Once he has accepted the new flavour and is eating only raw ground meat, the next step is to proceed to different minced meats, meat with ground bone, and, ideally, big pieces of bone and meat for him to chew (such as a chicken thigh).

I am assuming here that you have a healthy cat with a full set of teeth. If your cat is very old, toothless or ill, he may not manage to reach a stage where he eats such a fully natural diet. If, for instance, he will transition from tinned to minced meat, but refuses to eat the crunchy version with added bone, you may need to supplement his diet with a phosphate binder to ensure a natural mineral balance (see page 212). This may also be needed if you are feeding a raw meat diet to a cat with chronic kidney problems.

Discuss your desire to change diet with your veterinarian. A more appropriate diet may be what your cat needs, or perhaps the change will be too much. This calls for an individual assessment. If your vet is not able to guide you, see the chapter on page 37.

The perils of plastic

Avoid plastic food and water bowls, as plastic is known to contain harmful chemicals that can be absorbed with the food. Stainless-steel bowls often work well, but if you have a dog who is an enthusiastic eater, and find that the stainless-steel bowl is too noisy, or is light enough to go skating across the floor, ceramic bowls can be a nice alternative. Again, be aware of potentially toxic dyes in ceramics that are not intended for food. In many situations, using a bowl or plate designed for serving human food is a safer choice than a traditional dog or cat bowl.

FINAL WORDS ON FEEDING – WHICHEVER METHOD YOU CHOOSE

Trust your own judgement
Many of us have become so alienated from the simple task of putting food in front of dogs and cats that we worry about ensuring that they get everything they need. Yet we are fairly confident that we can feed our own children. Feeding a dog or a cat is in no way harder than feeding a human. There are a few things to consider, all of which have been covered in this chapter.

Throw away scales and guidelines
Whether you are feeding dry, tinned or raw, don't fret over tables and feeding guidelines.

Please don't weigh your dog's or cat's food. Give them what seems a reasonable amount that will be eaten in a single sitting. If they don't finish the meal, remove any leftovers and adjust the amount you give next time. Trust your own judgement and look at your animal. Is he too skinny, too fat or just about right? There are huge individual differences in metabolism, activity level, and so on. Any amount stated in a table is only a suggested estimate, and may be completely wrong for your particular dog or cat. If your pet ends up looking a bit too lean or a bit too round, add or remove about 20% of his food.

Of course, there are variations in body type, but a much more accurate method than weighing is assessing a dog's body score by placing a flat hand on his ribs, which you should be able to feel easily, but without them being visible. Excess fat on cats tends to droop under their bellies.

Look at your dog or cat rather than at standardised tables. Is his coat thick and glossy? Are his teeth and gums healthy? Does he have bad breath? Is he energetic and happy? Most of us trust our own judgement to ensure that our kids are happy and healthy, and I have never yet seen a measuring cup used to determine the amount of food a seven-year-old child should eat for dinner. However much pet food companies would like to sell you the idea, feeding a dog or cat is *not* rocket science.

Mix and match

In describing the three approaches to feeding (processed, home cooked and raw), I do not mean to imply that you need to pick one and stick to it. By all means mix and match as it suits you and your animal. No diet is ideal for all, and fundamentalism is rarely healthy, so feel free to experiment and find what suits you as well as your dog and/or cat.

If you are feeding primarily what the rest of the family is having for dinner, with an

Perfect portions

The correct meal size is :
• when your dog or cat has a stable body weight that suits their type
• When they finish their meal in one go
Please don't weigh the food or rely on tables or feeding guides. Use common sense as your guide

emphasis on the meat, it may be wise to keep a bag of good quality kibble, or a bag of frozen meat, for those pizza, porridge, soup or curry days when the leftovers aren't suitable.

A large meaty bone once or twice a week will be a welcome addition to any diet. If you are primarily feeding dry or tinned food, you can dramatically increase both the nutritional value and the flavour by adding select healthy leftovers from your own meals.

Some dog owners prefer to buy the cheapest kibble available and feed it half and half with proper fresh meat from the family household, as opposed to investing in the most expensive kibble for the higher content of animal protein.

It is often said that you should not feed raw meat together with anything else, as this will raise stomach pH, and increase the time it takes the food to pass through the digestive tract, potentially compromising digestion of the raw meat and bones. I can only say that I have been recommending raw feeding for more than 20 years, and have never seen a problem result from mixing diets.

It is probably best, if you feed both raw and dry, that you feed in separate meals rather than literally mix it together in the same bowl. My own dogs and cats eat a mixture of leftovers, good quality dry food and BARF.

No one way suits everyone: find yours.

Don't beat yourself up

If you have always fed your animals dry,

processed food and you feel overwhelmed by the idea of fundamentally changing what works for you, then don't. There are plenty of small steps that can make a big difference. Don't feel guilty about your choices, or fall into the trap of thinking that there is one perfect approach.

Maybe, having read this chapter, you will study the labels more and consider a better brand. Maybe you will more often supplement the diet with high quality leftovers such as human-grade meat. Remember, it is just food: yes, it is important, but it really isn't complicated. Do what works for you and your animals.

Who's your vet?

When I was 12 years old, I knew that I would be a vet. My decision was made at such a young age that I honestly don't even remember it as a conscious choice. It was just obvious.

After more than 25 years in veterinary practice, I am very aware of what a privileged life this is. Not just because of the animals, as one might think, but equally because I spend all day surrounded by people, colleagues and clients alike, who love animals. It takes a special kind of person to choose dirt and dog hair, to take on the obligation to come straight home from work every day, and to calculate pet sitters into any weekend or holiday plan.

A love of animals and the willingness to live with the practical and emotional upheavals that they bring, are not things that can be explained to those who don't share them. Furthermore, I have come to realize that the people who do share them are simply the nicest people, and I have had the pure luck to be able to surround myself with them.

I promise you that whoever your vet is, they have chosen their path in life because they share your love for animals.

An important ally

Because of the shorter lifespan of cats and dogs compared to humans, I am tempted to say that it is even more important that you find the right veterinarian for your animals than the right GP for yourself (although, by all means, do both). My point is simply that, sooner or later, you will need a vet.

A great vet can be invaluable in supporting you throughout your animals' lives, monitoring their health, and advising on how to keep them in top form. Maybe you are so experienced in their care that you don't need a veterinarian for lifestyle advice, or perhaps you rely on other sources of information, like your breeder, your friends, your dog trainer, social media interest groups ... or this book!

Even so, one day you will need a vet. Your dog may be involved in an accident or become ill. Even the healthiest (and luckiest) cat or dog, who manages to dodge both cars and germs, will grow old within a decade, and likely require extra support for the complaints of old age; maybe even euthanasia.

If you leave your choice of vet to chance or until the day you suddenly need one, you risk finding yourself and your animal in a vulnerable situation, without the support you deserve. Find out about the veterinarians in your area. Use routine visits as scouting missions to meet the vets, and ask a few well-chosen questions in order to determine who is for you and who you want to avoid.

This way, when (or if) the day comes when you rush through the door of the veterinary clinic with a seriously sick cat or dog, feeling sick with worry yourself, you will be met by someone who knows you and your animal, knows the animal's medical history, his lifestyle, and how he behaves when he is well. Someone who also understands how you like to do things, and who shares or at least respects your general approach to healthcare.

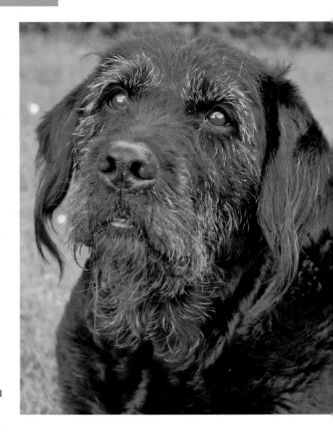

What makes a good veterinarian?

You want a vet, of course, who is good at their job, and who has a good bedside manner. There is more to it than that, however, and the right vet for your neighbour may not be the right vet for you.

Some people like to be told the story straight, while others prefer to have bad news broken to them gently. Some want to run every test, and need to know that no stone has been left unturned, while others are happier with a less invasive approach, and prefer to ensure maximum comfort for the patient. It is almost never the case that there is only one obvious way to proceed.

Much more commonly, there are choices to be made regarding tests and treatments – choices to be made in a partnership between you and your veterinarian. Do yourself a favour and find the right partner for this

important role. Know who you would go to if the need should arise tomorrow. Every day, someone tells me their story of feeling poorly supported at a difficult time. Maybe the veterinarian was rude to them (yes, it happens; I apologise on behalf of my chosen profession) about their choice of diet or some other lifestyle choice that they fundamentally disagreed about. Maybe they felt pressured into expensive or invasive procedures without properly understanding the expected outcome, or perhaps they felt that relevant treatments weren't discussed because of the animal's age or the vet's prejudice.

When carers and vets clash, as they sometimes do, it is not always the vet who is to blame, however. We are all different, and vets are people, too. For your own sake – and for the sake of your animal – find the right vet for you; *before* the day you really need one.

How to find the vet in your life

It is not uncommon to shop around, using whichever veterinary clinic is closest, cheapest, has the best parking, or has an available appointment at a convenient time. This is a great approach if you are still in the scouting phase, checking out the vets in your area and taking any opportunity to meet them.

Once you have found the right one, though, stay faithful. You may feel that it doesn't matter much where you go for simple things such as vaccinations, worming or small surgical procedures that anyone can do, and I agree, provided you are still searching for your family vet. But don't go back to the one you didn't very much trust because you are there for something simple. Take the opportunity to go to a different surgery, and ask about its ethos.

It is far too easy to shop around randomly throughout an animal's life, so that maybe four or five vets end up treating the same dog for ear infections, or the same cat for cystitis, without any of them realising that this is a recurrent problem that needs to be properly addressed. Consistent personal care is invaluable. Don't settle for less.

The vet-to-be interview

There are at least four important lifestyle choices that you will make for your dog or cat: diet, vaccinations, neutering and parasite control.

These topics are thoroughly discussed in the first section of this book, and I expect that you already know how you would like to approach some or all of these four areas. Whether you base your choices on hours of research or rely on intuition, your approach to these decisions (which every carer makes) reflects who you are and how you would like your dog or cat to live.

If you simply ask your vet (or unknowing applicant for the trusted position as your vet-to-be) what their recommendations are, it will be very easy to see if you are a good match. Does their approach match yours? Are they happy to enter into dialogue, and do they listen to and respect your point of view? If not, simply take your puppy or kitten elsewhere for the next booster or health check, and proceed to interview the next applicant in line.

At the time of writing this book, the 2010 WSAVA vaccination guidelines, though already nearly ten years old, are still so far from being universally implemented that this is my recommendation for a first vet-screening question: what is their recommended vaccination protocol, and do they do in-house titre testing? If they are not scientifically sound, updated and ethical in this area, where it is so easy for you to fact-check their answers (see the chapter on vaccination, page 42), do you want to rely on them in an emergency, when you have to trust their judgement?

I strongly recommend that you spend some time and energy on Project Find-the-Right-Vet-for-Us. Do the legwork early on, and you will have a trusted ally when you need one most.

Stress-free visits

Avoiding stress to an animal is, of course, always a goal in itself. Apart from that, though, there are plenty of practical reasons why all parties should make an effort to keep visits to the veterinarian as stress-free as possible.

A relaxed dog or cat is much easier to examine properly without the need for restraint or sedation. It is much easier to assess the gait, posture and general demeanour and wellbeing of an animal who isn't cowering and tense just from being at the vet's.

Nobody likes injections

In some countries, a visit to a veterinarian will almost always end in an injection. Okay, I admit that I may be exaggerating somewhat to prove my point, but it is almost as though custom dictates the routine injection to conclude the visit. If there is no injection, you clearly didn't need to come in the first place. Vets may subconsciously feel that, without an injection, they haven't really earned their fee.

If no other injection is justifiable, maybe a vitamin injection just to keep everyone satisfied?

If you recognise this pattern, whether you are a vet or an animal carer, I invite you to challenge it.

There is generally no reason why a course of antibiotics should be begun with an injection at the vets, only to be continued with tablets at home. Why not simply start the tablets straight away and forget the injection? This is, after all, how it is generally done when humans need antibiotics or other drugs from their GP.

If the treatment is so urgent that it actually calls for an injection, I suspect the patient should be hospitalised. This tradition of seemingly mandatory injections, where it exists, obviously does little to help dogs and cats relax at the vet's.

Where everybody knows your name

Limiting the use of injections is just one of many initiatives that can transform the dreaded veterinary clinic into an animal-friendly environment. Many clinics invite dog owners to drop by now and then for a friendly greeting or treat from the receptionist, so that, for your animal, the clinic's front door represents not the gates of hell but rather a familiar and friendly place to visit. If the clinic you use or plan to use is out of the way, this is an opportunity to take your dog into the waiting room for a quick hello if you ever go there to buy food, snacks, toys or other products.

Some clinics use pheromone diffusers to achieve an animal-friendly ambience. Some vets always apply a quick pheromone spray to the examination table before calling in the next feline patient. For more on the calming use of pheromones, see page 214. If your dog or cat

is apprehensive by nature or already affected by memories of past painful vet visits, a few doses of Rescue Remedy (see page 111) or of a calming supplement (see page 214) before you set off for a visit can sometimes make a big difference.

The annual health check

As the 'annual vaccination' visit that previously brought most dogs and cats to the vet once a year is no more (see the chapter on vaccination, page 42), is there any reason to take a healthy animal to see the vet every year?

Think of it this way: in terms of relative life expectancy, a health check every year for a dog or cat is the equivalent of every five to ten years for a human. A lot can happen in a year, added to which your dog or cat cannot tell you where it hurts. It is easy to miss small or gradual changes, but your veterinarian will be able to pick up on incipient problems, and advise on the best steps to prevent them developing.

An investment in the future

I suggest that you view the annual health check as a chance to ask all of the questions that may have occurred to you over the past year. Ask about behaviour, classes, pet sitters, parasite prevention, titre testing, diet, supplements, and so on. Your vet is a font of knowledge, and has an invaluable local network. Use her.

A thorough physical examination every year is a great investment. Depending on your animal's age and state of health, extra tests such as an evaluation of urine, stool or blood samples, may be relevant, too. On top of these obvious reasons for a visit, the fact that all three of you – patient, vet and carer – know each other will make a world of difference should the day come when you may have to face difficult decisions. Not only because it will feel better, but because your vet will be far better equipped to assess a dog or cat who is known to her; because she will know how you like to approach things, and because you will have faith in the person advising you.

My vet doesn't understand me

You may be reading this chapter thinking, 'That's all very well and good, but my vet just isn't like that.'

If you have a vet who is caught up in the old ways of feeling the need to justify a fee by pushing for some kind of injection or procedure, I suggest that you start by matching expectations. Declare from the outset that you are very happy to pay for their time, professional opinion and advice; you do not necessarily expect any action to take place today. There are many acute situations, that will most likely clear up with a little time (and perhaps a supplement or cream and some TLC), in which your vet may feel inclined to bring out the heavy drugs, just in case. There is pressure to treat because you showed up, and vets are aware that it doesn't look good if they do nothing and the condition worsens so that you return in a few days to get the drugs anyway, and have to pay for a second consultation.

Tell her, if this is how you feel, that you are just there to have it looked at, and are happy to see how it goes and come back again if needed.

Too often, in my opinion, animals are over-treated simply because the owners take them to the vet, and the vet feels pressure to do something. Just as often, animals who should have been seen by a vet are not because their owners fear she will jump on them with loaded syringes as soon as they get in the door.

Vets are well-educated people, generally simply keen to provide a good service, but they aren't mind-readers. It is your responsibility to either speak to your vet about your expectations, or, if you really don't find her approachable, to leave and find another vet who is.

If you live in the Australian outback, I admit that you may have a problem, but if, like most of us, you live within an hour's drive of several veterinary clinics, please don't just stick with the closest one and hope for the best. This is a relationship worth investing in, and an extra half hour's travel time is neither here nor there.

It's not a matter of someone being a bad vet. An extremely competent, capable and experienced vet, who comes recommended by lots of happy customers, will not be a good support for you if they fundamentally disagree with your way of doing things.

Visit Hubble and Hattie on the web: www.hubbleandhattie.com
hubbleandhattie.blogspot.co.uk
• Details of all books • Special offers • Newsletter • New book news

Vaccination

You may remember a time, not so many years ago, when it was common practice to repeatedly vaccinate our pets against every illness for which there was a vaccine.

First, it was every year, and then it changed to every second or third year (you can, in fact, still come across this recommendation today). The only rationale behind this practice was that no one really knew how long the protection from each vaccination lasted, or even considered that vaccination could cause side effects. The feeling was that, even if repeated vaccinations were, perhaps, not needed to maintain protection, and even if some vaccines didn't work very well, at least they couldn't hurt, and they did bring pets to the vet for regular check-ups.

Then came the discovery in the early 1990s that some cats develop fatal cancers at the injection site as a direct result of vaccination. This led to a new way of thinking about vaccines, and a concerted effort on the part of the veterinary community to establish, for the first time, the actual need for vaccination in dogs and cats, rather than simply relying on the recommendations of vaccine manufacturers.

The American Association of Feline Practitioners (AAFP) produced the very first veterinary vaccination guidelines in 1998, and, since then, veterinary experts have continued to release updated guidelines to inform both vets and the public about the safe and correct use of vaccines for dogs and cats. It is worth noting that these guidelines aim to minimise the number of vaccines given to each animal.

Vets today, therefore, have access to clear vaccination guidelines published by the world's leading experts in the field of dog and cat immunology: the Vaccination Guidelines Group of the World Small Animal Veterinary Association (WSAVA), that publishes global guidelines for both cats and dogs. It is a huge step forward for the health of our dogs and cats that these guidelines exist, so that we can use vaccines in a way that is based on scientific medical advice rather than mere assumption or commercial interests – and it falls to every vet to follow them.

I will explain these guidelines and their implications in detail over the following pages.

If your interest in vaccination is limited to its practical application, however, and all you want to know is what you should do, feel free to skip straight to the recommended vaccination programmes on pages 56 (dogs) and 57 (cats).

A time of ground-breaking changes

In my opinion as a vet, the fact that experts (independent veterinary immunologists) are now informing and guiding vets on the proper use of vaccination for dogs and cats is the greatest advance in small animal care in many decades. For far too long, vaccines were blindly administered without scientific justification.

Whilst this is an exciting time, however, it is also for many a confusing one, which is why I choose to go into some detail on this topic.

Old habits do, indeed, die hard, and during this period of transition, while the new guidelines are being implemented everywhere, we have a situation where animal owners may receive conflicting advice from different local veterinary practices, as some adjust their longstanding habits and traditions faster than others. In another decade (and I hope much sooner than that), this period of transition will surely have come to an end, and all vaccines will be administered in line with current medical knowledge.

In the meantime, the dedicated dog or cat owner may wish to ensure that they are up-to-date on the recent advances. I am here to help.

The period of transition

Our knowledge on this topic is still relatively new, and, frustratingly, it takes a long time for information to spread and change to occur.

As we go through this period of change, when old habits are superseded and new routines are established everywhere, many informed owners (like yourself) will meet with rules and restrictions based on old dogma.

It is simply a case of established regulations needing to catch up with the science, and you may find yourself in conversation with dog trainers, kennel owners, vets, exhibition officials or other dog or cat owners who are not yet fully updated on the new guidelines.

I hope that you will help spread the word, and insist that your animal is never given a vaccine he doesn't need.

Life-long protection

As a rule, the WSAVA guidelines mean that vaccination of adult dogs should now be considered a thing of the past (at least outside of areas where rabies and leptospirosis are endemic diseases). In fact, with optimal timing, a dog can achieve life-long protection through one single vaccination received as a puppy.

The jury is in

Please be aware that this is not a question of differing opinions. There is no ongoing debate between opposing points of view; there are simply vets who follow current scientific guidelines (written by groups of independent academic experts at the request of veterinary associations), and vets who, for whatever reason, have not yet updated their practice. The experts agree, and the guidelines are clear and widely available – albeit at odds, perhaps, with the commercial interests that have historically promoted over-vaccination.

It may also be important to emphasise that the information presented in this chapter is in no way an holistic or alternative view, but rather the *latest scientific advice at the time of publication*. While recommendations may evolve as we acquire more knowledge, the experts of the WSAVA's vaccination guidelines group are the scientific authority on this matter, and their latest document will always be your point of reference.

Please help spread the word to the

benefit of our cats and dogs. There is a list of references at the back of this book in case you ever need to document the information. Refer to the list, to the full version of the guidelines (available on the WSAVA website at www. wsava.org), and to this book as we help one another to protect dogs and cats from the ill-founded vaccination practices of the past.

Immunity

Immunity is a complex and deeply fascinating topic: don't forget that immunity involves much more than vaccination. We all know that the likelihood of our coming down with flu when someone sneezes in our direction at a bus stop depends on many other factors than merely whether or not we had a flu jab this year. The virulence of the particular virus, and the amount of exposure we receive are important factors, but so is whether you are otherwise healthy and have a high natural resistance because your immune system is strong. Are you sleeping well? Eating healthily? Or are you tired, stressed, and therefore highly susceptible?

Health doesn't primarily come out of a syringe. See also page 89 for lifestyle measures other than vaccination to protect cats in particular against infectious diseases.

Why vaccinate at all?

As new evidence of possible harm from needless vaccination continues to emerge, some animal carers have chosen to refrain from vaccinating their animals altogether. This could be a very dangerous development.

A dog or cat may indeed live a long, healthy life without a single vaccine. This is due partly to a phenomenon known as herd immunity. If a large enough proportion (around 75%) of individuals in an area are protected against a disease, the disease cannot spread, and, as a consequence, even the unvaccinated individuals won't become ill. If the majority of animals are unvaccinated,

So, when?

It is important to minimise the number of vaccinations given to each dog or cat. We do this in two ways. First by vaccinating only against illnesses that are both clearly serious enough to justify the risk of vaccination and prevalent enough in the local environment to present a real risk of infection. Second, we avoid repeating these vaccines unnecessarily. Titre testing is a great tool for checking the duration of immunity in individual animals.

however, a very different situation emerges, and epidemics can occur.

I certainly see dogs and cats who have been vaccinated at the wrong time or with the wrong vaccine, at great detriment to their health. I have also, when working as a young vet in a part of London where many dogs were left unvaccinated, cared for puppies who were extremely ill from parvovirus, and I have watched some of them die.

Knowing that their suffering was completely preventable made it so much worse. Vaccines can save lives and certainly still have a role to play. This is a complicated topic that cannot be reduced to a position of being for or against vaccination. Vaccination isn't inherently good or bad. In order to understand how to use vaccines in a safe and beneficial manner, we must understand which diseases warrant vaccination, and how often the vaccines against those diseases should be repeated to maintain protection. We must use vaccines rationally and responsibly. After many decades of fumbling in the dark, we are finally getting there.

How vaccines work

Through vaccination, dogs and cats are exposed to either killed or weakened ('attenuated') disease material. This is done so that the animal, by being exposed without becoming ill, produces antibodies against the illness in question, and via these antibodies and the ability to produce them, will be protected if ever exposed to this particular disease.

Two types of vaccine

There are two main types of vaccine: killed vaccines and live attenuated vaccines. Most of the core vaccines in common use are live vaccines, but killed vaccines are also used for both cats and dogs: allow me to quickly outline (in a somewhat simplistic form) the main differences.

Live attenuated (weakened) vaccines

- Fewer side effects than killed vaccines

- Longer duration of protection (in most cases lifelong)

- In the absence of maternal antibodies, one vaccination will provide full protection. (Repeated vaccination of puppies and kittens under 16 weeks of age is done only because of the risk that maternal antibodies will block the vaccine. Adult animals and puppies or kittens who are 16 weeks or older need one shot only to be protected)

- A vaccine provides protection after three to four days

- Parvovirus, distemper and hepatitis are examples of live vaccines for dogs

- Panleukopenia, herpesvirus and calicivirus are live vaccines given to cats

Killed vaccines

- Higher risk of side effects because of the adjuvants (a substance that enhances the body's immune response to an antigen) added to killed vaccines

- The initial vaccination generally requires two vaccines given three to six weeks apart, regardless of the animal's age. (More may be needed if the animal is under 16 weeks old at the time of the initial vaccination, as maternal antibodies may block the vaccine. If the first of the series is blocked by maternal antibodies, the second shot won't work either)

- The effect of killed vaccines is relatively shortlived. Some require annual revaccination

- The vaccine series doesn't provide protection until one week after the second vaccine (at least three weeks after the first of the two vaccinations)

- Rabies is a killed vaccine, but it is so powerful that it differs in several of the above points, and in practice is used more like a live vaccine. Leptospirosis is a good example of a killed vaccine in use for dogs

Can vaccines do harm?

Vaccines can absolutely do harm; no one disputes this fact. Unintended side effects are a risk we take whenever we introduce a drug into the body, and the potential for putting undue strain on the immune system by subjecting it to vaccines has long been well established.

It is always a matter of weighing the benefits against the risks. There are several ways in which a vaccination may do harm. Cats, for example, may develop cat flu if they inhale or lick up minute amounts of cat flu vaccine accidentally left on the fur at the injection site. A small percentage of cats even develop fatal cancers as a direct consequence of leukaemia or rabies vaccination.

Some dogs and cats also suffer an immediate anaphylactic reaction after a vaccination. Symptoms of this may be redness of the skin and eyes, swelling, and difficulty breathing. The vet will treat the anaphylaxis as a matter of urgency, and deaths from anaphylaxis are extremely rare. This is, however, the reason you should not leave your dog or cat unattended for the first few hours after a vaccine is given. Anaphylactic reactions are easy to observe and fairly easy to treat, although urgency is crucial.

Although all vets see these reactions now and then, and although they are clear and dramatic when they happen, acute anaphylactic reactions are in many ways of less concern than the possibly more long-term chronic side effects of vaccinations.

It is very difficult to establish a causal link to vaccination when dogs and cats develop epilepsy, allergies or thyroid, kidney or autoimmune disease, but these are, in fact, all conditions that we now know may occur as a direct consequence of vaccination. Studies have also shown that more serious illness appears more often in the first three months after vaccination than at any other period in an animal's life. Although everyone agrees that negative vaccine reactions are grossly under-reported, it is impossible to get a clear idea of the true extent of the negative health implications of vaccination.

It is said that small breeds are more at risk of vaccine-adverse reactions than larger breeds; that combination vaccines cause more problems than single vaccines, and that killed vaccines (that is, vaccines against leptospirosis and rabies in dogs, and leukaemia and rabies in cats) cause far more side effects than other vaccines. Suffice to say that there is certainly evidence to back up the WSAVA's vaccine guidelines report when it cautions that any vaccine given to any animal poses a risk, and that the side effects may not cause disease for months or even years after the responsible vaccine was administered. The

Caution!

If your dog or cat has clearly reacted adversely to a vaccine before, please don't vaccinate him again. The not-uncommon approach of administering a steroid dose at the time of vaccination to individuals who are known to suffer acute side effects after vaccination is, in my opinion, an example of the worst imaginable kind of poor judgement. Vaccination should be used with caution in all individuals, and not at all in those who are particularly sensitive to vaccinosis (the ill effects of vaccination).

WSAVA report concludes that it is therefore important to minimise the number of vaccines given to any individual animal.

How do we protect animals from vaccine damage?

We protect animals against vaccine side effects (vaccinosis) primarily by making sure that they only get the vaccines that they really need. Only vaccinate against core diseases, unless there are clear reasons why your particular animal needs non-core vaccines, and use titre testing to check the duration of the immunity in order to avoid unnecessary boosters.

We also protect animals from the risks of vaccine damage by ensuring that only healthy animals are vaccinated. The American veterinary immunologist Jean Dodds furthermore recommends that we not only avoid vaccinating pregnant and lactating bitches, but also avoid vaccinating a bitch when she is in heat, and for a period of 30 days before and after her season. Dr Dodds also recommends that, as far as possible, we avoid giving multiple vaccines at the same time, and avoid vaccinating geriatric animals altogether.

Titre testing – the answer to (almost) everything

A titre test is a cheap, easy and simple way to check if your dog or cat remains protected by the last core vaccine, whenever this was given.

Your vet or veterinary nurse will take a small blood sample, which is then checked for specific antibodies. Your vet may send the sample to a lab, of course, but the test can now be done using a simple test kit, and takes just half an hour, so more and more veterinary practices offer this as an in-house service, which greatly reduces the cost.

To my mind, it is indefensible to revaccinate an adult animal against core diseases without first doing a titre test to establish if the animal already has antibodies against the disease in question (see page 53 on the definition of core diseases). The presence or absence of antibodies against a given disease provides a clear yes/no answer to the question of whether or not the animal is protected. There is no degree of protection; nor is it relevant to refer to levels of antibodies. It is an easy, all-or-nothing situation.

A **positive** titre means that antibodies are present, and, therefore, that the animal is still protected. There will be some false-negative results in animals that do not have circulating antibodies at the time of testing, but whose white blood cells still retain the ability to produce them. This is because immunity happens through several mechanisms. We cannot measure cell-mediated protection, only the antibodies present in the blood at a given point, so titre testing may miss some animals who are actually still protected. An animal who tests positive, however, is definitely protected, and will gain nothing from further vaccines: if protection is still there, all you would get from a booster are the side effects.

It should be very clear, then, that revaccinating in the presence of antibodies is pure madness. Revaccinating an adult dog or cat without first checking for antibodies exposes the animal to unnecessary risk, and simply makes no sense.

What diseases can we titre test for?

We currently have reliable titre tests for parvovirus, distemper and hepatitis in dogs, and for panleukopenia in cats. Titre testing for cat flu (calicivirus and herpesvirus) is available but, according to WSAVA experts, should not be considered reliable. While there seems to be some disagreement among immunologists on this point, I tend to follow WSAVA's advice, and so I currently recommend against relying on titre testing to assess immunity against cat flu.

We can test reliably for protection against rabies, but rabies vaccination is generally a matter of adhering to legislation, and in this context a titre test is still not accepted in lieu of a vaccination certificate. This will surely change in the future.

For the suggested timing of titre tests, see page 48 as well as the vaccination programmes on pages 56 (dogs) and 57 (cats).

Is titre testing reliable?

In the past, experts have discussed what level of antibodies constitutes protective levels, and advocates of the status quo approach to vaccination have tried to cast doubt on the reliability of titre testing (old habits die hard, and vaccination is, undeniably, big business). This doubt has now been settled, and today experts agree that titre testing (including the use of in-house titre test kits) is, as the chair of the WSAVA's Vaccination Guideline Group puts it, 'the new revolutionary tool in veterinary medicine.'

According to WSAVA guidelines, in the case of parvovirus, distemper and hepatitis there is total correlation between the presence of circulating antibodies and protection against disease. If the animal can produce specific antibodies against the core diseases, it means that the vaccine worked, and the animal is fully protected. The size of the titre (how many antibodies are found in a blood test) is of no significance. If there are any antibodies at all, the vaccine has done its job and the cat or dog is protected against the disease in question.

Put another way, an animal with a *low* positive titre is every bit as protected as an animal with a *high* positive titre. It is my experience that there is a lot of confusion about this. Dog and cat owners (and indeed vets and their staff) sometimes suffer from the misconception that a higher titre makes it more likely that the result will stay positive for years to come, or that the result of a titre test is merely a random 'snapshot' in time, and that protection might therefore no longer be present two weeks after the day of the test.

If you hear these opinions, rest assured that they are based on a misunderstanding. Studies have shown that immunity is lifelong in 98% of puppies following puppy vaccination alone, which means that immunity against core diseases simply does not wane in the overwhelming majority of cases, and will not (ever!) need 'boosting.' 'Booster' is, in fact, an unfortunate word to use in connection with core vaccines, as it implies a gradual decline of immunity over time, which we now know is not expected to happen.

The WSAVA stresses that titre testing is not only reliable, but also constitutes a higher standard of veterinary practice. This is not simply a matter of striving to reduce the

incidence of vaccine side effects; rather, it reflects a core principle of good medicine: that we should never perform a procedure (in this case a vaccination) without first establishing that it is indicated and in the patient's best interest. I second this point, and would even go so far as to recommend using a pet clinic's adherence to WSAVA vaccination guidelines (including the use of in-house titre testing) as an easy way to tell the good from the bad. Good medicine is just good medicine.

How often should titre tests be repeated?

There can be little doubt that the current WSAVA recommendation of repeating a titre test every three years for adult dogs is applicable only for the current period of transition, as we move from frequently repeated vaccinations to the future approach of vaccinating only puppies. Everyone apparently needs to see for themselves that immunity does indeed last – and perhaps vets need to feel reassured that their services are still required.

In my opinion, there is no pressing need for repeated titre testing of adult animals unless it is required for the dog or cat to be accepted into boarding kennels, training classes, shows, and so on. The fact remains that, once achieved, a positive titre against the core diseases is never expected to reduce. The important titre test is certainly the first one, which can be done at any time, but is ideally scheduled for one to two months after the last puppy or kitten vaccine, meaning at around the age of five to six months. If a titre test is positive at this time, it proves that the individual has a well-functioning immune system, and that the puppy or kitten vaccination has worked. In most cases, further vaccination can then be forgotten about.

As I have repeated several times, studies show that, once a puppy has been immunised against the core diseases, immunity can be expected to last for many

Titre testing

The WSAVA recommends that all dogs and cats are titre tested at five to six months of age, following the puppy/kitten vaccines, and that titre tests are then repeated every three years until the age of 10 (for dogs) or 15 (for cats), after which annual testing is suggested.

years, and probably for life. Therefore, the reasonable expectation is that a titre test at any point in said puppy's life will be positive, and that a positive titre will remain so for many, many years.

The WSAVA currently recommends that titre testing is done every three years, and suggests increasing this to annual testing for dogs over the age of 10 and cats over the age of 15, who, theoretically, could lose immunity as their immune systems weaken with age. The esteemed American veterinary immunologist Dr Jean Dodds takes the opposite view, suggesting instead that titre testing is discontinued altogether for elderly animals. In her view, regardless of the result of the test (that is, even if the test is negative), old animals should not be vaccinated, as they will be weaker and more likely to suffer vaccination side effects.

A test for life

Once a puppy has responded to vaccination and become immune to parvovirus, distemper and hepatitis, this immunity is expected to last for life. A titre test will tell you quickly and clearly whether your dog is still protected against these core diseases. Never let anyone revaccinate your adult dog against any of the core diseases without first insisting on a titre test.

The homeopathic remedy Thuja

As a further precaution against vaccine side effects, I routinely administer the homeopathic remedy Thuja at the time of vaccination. Your vet can easily give a drop or pill directly into the mouth of your dog or cat at the time of the injection. If your vet doesn't do this, you can give it yourself. In this case, I recommend giving Thuja 30C or 200C once on the day before the vaccination, twice on the day (before and after the vet visit), and once on the following day.

The intention is simply to surround the vaccination with Thuja, by giving this before and after the vaccination. The ideal amount is impossible to establish – one dose at the vet's is probably sufficient – and the protective effect of Thuja is hard to document. Being a homeopathic preparation, however, it has no side effects, and, having practiced homeopathy for many years, I have seen enough cases of obvious vaccine damage being cured by Thuja that I do recommend its use as a preventative: it really can't hurt.

For more about homeopathy, see pages 117 and 218.

Homeopathic vaccines

There is no such thing as homeopathic vaccination. There are homeopathic remedies made from disease material, known as nosodes, which are sometimes used to prevent disease. Nosodes don't produce an antibody response, so they cannot reasonably be referred to as vaccines.

One of the fathers of veterinary homeopathy in the UK, Christopher Day, whom I had the great fortune to have as a teacher, published a study in 1987 that clearly demonstrated the effect of kennel cough nosode during an outbreak of kennel cough in a boarding shelter. I have no doubt that nosodes can prevent disease – in fact, in the case of kennel cough, I am quite sure that the nosode works better than the vaccine. I seriously doubt, however, that the dog or cat receiving a nosode can store the information. I therefore recommend the use of nosodes only in situations of known imminent exposure, that is, during an epidemic.

Giving a nosode (or a preparation of mixed nosodes) monthly, every three to six months or, indeed, on any set schedule, as is sometimes recommended, simply does not convince me. It would require the dog's or cat's system somehow remembering the information contained in the nosode if exposed to a disease months after the nosode was administered, and I have seen no evidence that this is likely to happen. For this reason, I advocate using a minimal (but effective) programme of well-timed conventional vaccinations as recommended by the WSAVA (preferably with homeopathic support; see page 49), and I do not support the routine use of nosodes against core diseases. Indeed, as discussed in this chapter, once titre testing shows that the puppy vaccines are effective, your puppy needs no further protection, and the use of nodoses against core diseases is not relevant (the situation for kittens is slightly more complicated).

If, however, there is ever an outbreak in your local area (typically, this would be of parvovirus or kennel cough for dogs, and cat flu for cats), do give your animal a daily dose of the relevant nosode (preferably not a mixture of several nosodes) for as long as the acute threat persists.

Cats suffer from a number of contagious diseases, for many of which we don't even have conventional vaccines, so situations certainly may arise that warrant consulting a homeopathic vet for advice on nosode protection if there is known illness in other cats in the household or local environment.

Puppies and kittens – timing is everything
Puppies and kittens get what is known as passive immunity through their mother's first milk (the colostrum) during the first 24 hours of life. Assuming that the mother was vaccinated and therefore has protective antibodies against a range of diseases, these antibodies are transferred to the young through the colostrum immediately after birth.

The level of these passively-acquired (so-called because they were not produced by the puppy's or kitten's own immune systems) maternal antibodies drops constantly until they finally provide no further protection, generally when the puppy or kitten is between eight and 16 weeks old. This age variation presents a big problem, as the time when the maternal antibodies drop away is precisely the right time to vaccinate the puppy. There will even be considerable variation between littermates as to when their maternal antibodies fall away.

Maternal antibodies act as a first line of defence, neutralising the disease matter that is the active ingredient in a vaccine, and so preventing it from having any effect. This is the reason why puppy and kitten vaccines are given as a series of vaccinations: we simply don't know when the level of maternal antibodies for each pup or kitten will be sufficiently low to allow the vaccine to work. We only know that, by the age of four months (16 weeks), all interference from maternal antibodies will have ceased for all puppies and kittens. In some 16-week-old animals, however, it will have dropped away only very recently, whilst, for others, it may have been absent for two months.

A single live vaccine given at 16 weeks will provide lasting immunity. Vaccines given before this age may or may not work, depending on the level of maternal antibodies in each puppy. For fear of leaving vulnerable puppies and kittens unprotected, we generally begin vaccinating a month or two before the 16-week mark; hence the need for a repeated vaccination at 16 weeks, in case the earlier ones were blocked by maternal antibodies. No matter how well we time the puppy vaccine, there will always be a window of susceptibility,

Belt-and-braces

A puppy responds to only one vaccination against the core diseases (parvovirus, distemper and hepatitis). When we give two or three in the so-called puppy series, it is purely because we don't know when each puppy is ready to be vaccinated. He will never respond to more than one of them.

during which the puppy is unprotected (when the passive immunity provided through the colostrum no longer affords protection until the time when the vaccine starts working). This cannot be avoided. We aim to make this window as small as possible, and for the rest we take comfort in the fact that, in most environments, puppies are protected by herd immunity (meaning that diseases are not rampant because a majority of animals are immune; see page 44).

The fact that a window of susceptibility inevitably exists must never be used as an argument for isolating a puppy until after vaccination – the general recommendation a couple of decades ago, but which has absolutely no merit. Puppies should attend puppy classes, meet other dogs, and generally be allowed to explore the world freely (also see page 11).

When to start vaccinating puppies and kittens
The WSAVA recommends ...
When titre testing is not used (see page 48) and multiple vaccines are therefore given as a puppy or kitten series, the WSAVA guidelines recommend that puppies receive a first core vaccine at eight to nine weeks of age; that this vaccine is repeated three to four weeks later, and again when the puppy is at least 16 weeks old. This means that each puppy receives the core vaccines three times each.

Of course, a puppy or kitten will respond to only one of these injections; specifically, the first one given after his maternal antibodies cease to provide protection. Vaccines given while the maternal antibodies are still present will be blocked by them, and vaccines repeated after a vaccine has already immunised the puppy will have no effect at all. Only one vaccine will work.

... but I think we should also consider ...
For most puppies and kittens, 12 weeks is probably a good age for the first vaccination

against core diseases. This should be followed by a second shot at 16 weeks, and ideally a titre test at 20 weeks. If the test is positive, chances are your pet is protected for life – and certainly for many years to come. Some young animals will run out of protective maternal antibodies before 12 weeks, so may benefit from receiving the first vaccine earlier. This could include puppies who have not received their mother's first milk, or kittens whose mothers were never vaccinated. In these cases, starting vaccination at eight weeks or perhaps even earlier may be preferable.

It may be that most puppies are ready to receive their first vaccine at or around eight weeks of age. If the puppy or kitten series is started at eight weeks (and titre testing is not used), your animal will need two further shots, given at 12 and 16 weeks, to make certain that he is covered through the first months of life, and ensure that no maternal antibodies interfere with the last vaccine given.

... because of this common case of bad timing
We now know that the process of vaccination has such a potent effect that the immune system cannot function optimally for a short time afterwards. The defences are down, so to speak, for about a week; specifically from day three to day ten after the vaccine is given. This is a general fact that applies to humans and animals alike, regardless of the type of vaccine given.

The immune system is distracted by the job of processing the vaccine, meaning that the individual is left more generally susceptible for a short while. This is rarely a problem in itself, but it certainly suggests that for a breeder to have puppies or kittens vaccinated shortly before sending them off to their new owners is very poor timing indeed.

There is probably no other period in their entire lives when young pups or kittens are more in need of an optimally-functioning immune system than during the first few days of settling into a completely new environment. In addition to the considerations discussed above regarding the ideal age to vaccinate a given animal, also remember that he should not be exposed to a new environment during the sensitive period (day three to day ten) following any vaccination.

For instance, if puppies are sold at eight weeks, it is far better for the informed breeder to leave it to the new owners to have them vaccinated after they have become accustomed to their new environment. Careful timing of the first vaccine can prevent many cases of sick puppies and kittens, whether from conjunctivitis, sneezing, diarrhoea or other acute infections contracted in the first days with their new families.

If you are waiting to pick up your puppy or kitten, make sure you discuss this with the breeder. Maybe they are fully informed; maybe you can help them get there. If they are not yet quite ready to move on from 'how things have always been done,' I suggest you firmly request that your particular puppy or kitten is *not* vaccinated when the litter is taken to the vet for the first health check and vaccination.

A veterinary health check of a full litter is generally a scene of fun and chaos as the puppies explore the room and the vet and breeder frantically try to identify which puppy gets which micro-chip, worming pill, vaccine, and so on. If your puppy is not to be vaccinated but other puppies in the litter are, I highly recommend that you ask your breeder to attach a ribbon to his collar, put him in a (leopard-print) coat, or unmistakeably mark him some other way as the one not to be vaccinated. Without this precaution, mistakes easily happen for the simple reason that puppies don't stay still.

When I give talks on the topic of vaccination, I frequently meet breeders who worry that no one will buy unvaccinated puppies and, equally frequently, puppy buyers who are convinced that no breeder will sell a puppy to them if they insist that he isn't vaccinated before they take him home. My experience is that all these fears are completely unfounded. People listen if you explain your reasons and document your viewpoint. In this, as in all vaccine matters, refer to the WSAVA guidelines and the other references listed at the back of this book. Some breeders have taken to selling unvaccinated puppies at eight weeks together with a copy of the original version of this book (published in Danish) in lieu of the first vaccination: a nice way to ensure that new owners are fully informed, and to show that the vaccination was postponed as a result of research, rather than due to neglect or a desire to cut costs.

Using titre testing to determine the optimal timing of the puppy vaccination

There is a solution (a very elegant solution, indeed) to the problem that we don't know exactly when the puppy's mother's antibodies have left his system, so that he can respond to vaccination.

We systematically give ineffective vaccines to all puppies because we don't know when each puppy is ready to be vaccinated. Instead, we could simply find out. The platinum standard of puppy care, then, is surely this: instead of blindly carpet-bombing your puppy's immune system because we don't know when he is ready to respond to vaccination, let's find out through titre testing.

Timing is everything ...

However you, your breeder, and your vet choose to plan the timing of the core vaccines for your pup, the one approach that must be avoided is giving the last puppy vaccine before he is 16 weeks old, without titre testing to check that protection has been achieved.

A titre test measures specific antibodies in the blood. If an unvaccinated, eight-week-old puppy tests positive, the fact that there are antibodies present in his blood tells us that his mother's antibodies are still protecting him, and that he cannot yet be vaccinated. Simply test him again in two to four weeks and vaccinate him when the titre test turns negative. In this way, he will need only a single vaccine against the core diseases (parvovirus, distemper and hepatitis; see page 56).

Vaccines are for healthy animals only

Only a healthy animal can respond appropriately to vaccination. This is reflected in the instruction sheet accompanying vaccines, which clearly states that the product must only be administered to healthy animals. This should be taken very literally.

If your dog or cat shows any symptoms – any signs of being under the weather – postpone the vaccine. It goes without saying that chronically ill animals should not be vaccinated. If your elderly cat suffers from failing kidneys or an overactive thyroid, or if your dog has asthma, epilepsy, cancer, allergies or any other long-term illness, then they are clearly not healthy, and it should be seriously considered whether a vaccine may be detrimental to their health.

The same goes for any animal receiving medication, particularly the immunosuppressive medication given to dogs and cats suffering from autoimmune or allergic disease. Pregnant bitches and queens should also not be vaccinated.

Core and non-core vaccines

The WSAVA vaccination guidelines divide vaccines into two groups: core vaccines and non-core vaccines. Core vaccines are those that should be given to all animals. For dogs, the core vaccines are against distemper, parvovirus and hepatitis. For cats, the core vaccines are panleukopenia (also called cat

parvovirus), herpesvirus and calicivirus (two of the causes of cat flu).

Non-core vaccines should never be given routinely. They must be given only when specific factors in the dog's or cat's lifestyle, geographical location, or other circumstances put them at particular risk. The non-core vaccines in common use in many countries are kennel cough and leptospirosis for dogs, and chlamydia and leukaemia for cats.

'Just to be safe'

I sometimes meet both colleagues and clients who seem to be under the impression that core vaccines constitute the 'basic package,' and that non-core vaccines are included in the deluxe vaccine package for the extra-discerning owner. This is completely wrong. The WSAVA makes it very clear that one of the main aims of the guidelines is minimising the use of non-core vaccines, by ensuring that they are given only when they are truly indicated. If everyone benefited from them, they wouldn't have been classified as *non-core* vaccines.

To put it simply, assume that your animal should receive core vaccines only. Those of you who are tempted to include the non-core vaccines 'just to be safe,' please understand that the recommendation of the experts who classified these vaccines as non-core was that, in the absence of compelling reasons to give them, they *should be avoided* precisely 'to be safe.' Non-core vaccines are for specific animals whose lives, for whatever reason, are deemed to be at greater risk. For everyone else, the risk of the non-core vaccine is not outweighed by its benefits.

Non-core vaccines are, by definition, those that do not benefit the general dog and cat population in most areas.

Rabies

Generally speaking, vaccinating pet animals against rabies is not a matter of protecting the

Core Matters

How often should an adult dog have a booster vaccine? The answer, in most cases, is never. The WSAVA states that, once a vaccine has immunised a puppy against the core diseases, in 98% of cases this protection will last for many years and probably for life. Yes, non-core vaccines need to be repeated annually, but the fact that these are classified as non-core means that most dogs don't need them at all.

animals, but rather of protecting humans from exposure to rabies infection. In many parts of America, rabies vaccination is mandatory. Where it is not, but where rabies is seen in any species, it may still be considered a core vaccine. In Australia, New Zealand and Europe, rabies vaccination is only relevant for dogs and cats who travel between countries. It is entirely a matter of fulfilling the legal requirements to cross international borders.

In this situation, I strongly recommend vaccinating only to fulfil the legal requirements; if you have no immediate travel plans, don't let your animal have this vaccine, and never give it routinely to young puppies and kittens. Don't keep the rabies vaccination up to date just in case you might one day decide to take your animal on holiday with you. Unless you travel very regularly or impulsively, it is far better to wait till the day approaches, and only then get the vaccine. Provided you have three weeks' warning of a trip abroad, this method is ideal, and may save your animal one or more rabies vaccines over a lifetime.

All evidence indicates that the actual duration of immunity following a rabies vaccine is much longer than the current legal validity of three years. I hope that regulations will be changed in the future to allow a positive rabies titre test to take the place of a vaccination certificate. If your dog or cat needs a rabies vaccine, make sure that it is not given at the

same time as any other vaccine. It is much safer to space out the vaccines by leaving at least two or three weeks between shots. Yes, it is certainly worth the extra trip to the veterinary clinic.

VACCINATION OF DOGS

The core vaccines for dogs are parvovirus, distemper and hepatitis.

Parvovirus: core live vaccine
Parvovirus causes explosive bloody diarrhoea. Affected animals quickly become dehydrated and, even with hospitalisation and intensive treatment, some will die. The virus can survive for a long time in the environment, so infection can spread, even without direct contact.

Distemper: core live vaccine
Distemper is a serious disease affecting the gastrointestinal tract, the airways, and the nervous system. It has, thanks to vaccination, become very rare in many countries, where younger vets may never have even seen a case.

Hepatitis (also referred to as adenovirus): core live vaccine
Hepatitis is a contagious disease of the liver. Symptoms include fever, vomiting and abdominal pain. Like distemper, it has become very rare in many countries, thanks to vaccination.

Leptospirosis: non-core killed vaccine
Leptospirosis symptoms range from mild unspecific disease to fatal kidney failure. When caught early, the disease is easily treatable with penicillin. Leptospirosis is a zoonosis (meaning that humans can contract it, too), but it is very difficult to find cases where humans and dogs have caught it from each other. Humans at risk of leptospirosis are primarily those employed on fish farms or

working in sewers; not dog owners.

This is classified as a non-core vaccine by the WSAVA. It is a relatively rare illness in most European countries, as it affects primarily tropical regions. On top of this, the WSAVA describes the leptospirosis vaccine as comparatively ineffective, and associated with a high risk of side effects. In many situations the potential benefit of the vaccine is simply not worth the risk.

The reason for its lack of effect is that there are more than 200 different types of leptospirosis, and the current vaccine recently went from including two to now covering four of these. Giving the leptospirosis vaccine is therefore no assurance that your dog won't catch the disease. I would not recommend this vaccine unless your dog is particularly at risk. I would never consider giving this vaccine to my own dogs, and I remain particularly worried about small breeds receiving it. As mentioned, the WSAVA has classified it as a non-core vaccine, meaning that it should not be given routinely. Some experts even recommend against its use in any circumstances, while others merely stress that it should not be used in dogs who live in cities, and should be restricted to dogs who hunt and who live in rural areas in regions (tropical climates) where this disease is endemic.

If, for some reason, you choose to let your dog have this vaccine, he will need two shots initially, followed by an annual booster (as this is a killed vaccine; see page 45).

Kennel cough: non-core live vaccine
Kennel cough is an infection of the upper airways that can be caused by a combination of factors and disease agents. You could say that it's the canine equivalent of having a throat infection or a common cold. It may require the patient to stay home and take it easy for a week or two, but the vast majority of cases require no other treatment than some rest and TLC. Severely weakened or very

---

WSAVA says ...

'The leptospirosis vaccine can be associated with adverse reactions. This vaccine should only be given if there is a real risk ... This product is associated with as many or more adverse reactions than occur from any other vaccine ... [and] is the one least likely to provide adequate and prolonged protection ... Leptospirosis may be relatively rare in your geographical area, so it's also worth asking your veterinary surgeon if he/she has recently seen any confirmed cases locally. If not, and your dog does not lead a lifestyle that carries a risk of exposure, you may decide not to vaccinate against leptospirosis ... Vaccination against leptospirosis should be restricted to use in geographical areas where a significant risk of exposure has been established.'

From Vaccination Guidelines for New Puppy Owners, *published by the World Small Animal Veterinary Association, 2013*

---

old individuals may suffer complications that require antibiotic treatment, but this is the rare exception.

For two reasons – namely, that this is generally a harmless disease, and that the vaccine is not very effective – there seems to be little sense in vaccinating. This is reflected in the fact that the WSAVA does not classify this as a core vaccine, meaning that it does not recommend it for routine use. In fact, more than one member of the WSAVA's vaccination guidelines group has publicly stated that the kennel cough vaccine doesn't work at all. Kennel cough is simply not a disease we can vaccinate effectively against: not surprising, really, as we are talking about a common cold.

Some dog trainers and some boarding kennels require dogs to have received a kennel cough vaccine. This is the most common reason for dog owners to request it. On the other hand, some dog trainers and boarding kennels do not admit dogs who have had the kennel cough vaccine because of the risk of shedding from a live vaccine (meaning that your dog could catch kennel cough from the vaccine or infect others). Make sure to check with your kennel beforehand. If you choose to give this vaccine; it must be repeated annually while relevant. It differs from other vaccines in that it is given into the nose rather than by injection. This can be an unpleasant and threatening experience for some dogs.

Rabies: killed vaccine
Use of rabies vaccination depends on your geographical region (see page 54). Rabies vaccination is non-core in Australia, New Zealand, and much of Europe, where it is only relevant for animals travelling abroad.

If your dog needs a rabies vaccine, make sure to give it at a different time than any other vaccines to minimise the risk of side effects. See more about rabies on page 53.

RECOMMENDED VACCINATION PROGRAMME FOR DOGS

The puppy series
(1) The three core vaccines – parvovirus, distemper and hepatitis – are given as a combination vaccine twice, at ages 12 and 16 weeks (or three times, at ages eight, 12 and 16 weeks).

If there is an outbreak of parvovirus in the local area, if the puppy did not receive colostrum, or if the mother was never vaccinated, it may be preferable to start vaccinating at eight weeks, or possibly even earlier. In this case, three puppy vaccines given four weeks apart will be needed (at eight, 12 and 16 weeks of age).

Alternatively, it is possible, by titre testing the puppy prior to vaccination, to ensure full protection from a single, perfectly-timed puppy vaccination.

Checking that the puppy series worked
(2) Titre test four weeks after the last puppy vaccine, at around 20 weeks of age to ensure that the puppy series has indeed provided lasting protection. If this titre test is positive, your puppy is protected, in most cases for many years, and possibly for life. If the test is negative, vaccinate again, preferably with a different product. A small percentage of dogs are so-called non-responders, and will never produce antibodies from vaccination. We have no way of knowing whether they are still protected through cellular mechanisms.

The years ahead
(3) You may choose to titre test every three to four years to demonstrate that your dog is still protected against the core diseases. This is necessary if boarding kennels, exhibition admittance or training courses require proof of lasting protection.

Other (non-core) vaccines
You may choose to vaccinate annually against kennel cough while this is relevant (typically, when boarding kennels or dog trainers demand it).

If you live in an area where rabies is endemic and vaccination is therefore a legal requirement, or if you travel abroad with your dog, he will need vaccination against rabies.

Other vaccines are not recommended for routine use. Read more under kennel cough, leptospirosis and rabies in this chapter.

VACCINATION OF CATS

The core vaccines for cats are feline panleukopenia, herpesvirus, and calicivirus.

Panleukopenia: core live vaccine
This is a very serious disease, causing high

fever with diarrhoea and vomiting. Most infected cats will not survive. The virus is very stable and can survive in the environment, which means that direct contact is not needed to spread the disease.

Cat flu (herpesvirus and calicivirus): core live vaccines

Cat flu is a general term for a range of infectious illnesses affecting the airways of cats. Symptoms include fever, sneezing and discharge from the nose and eyes.

The two most common causes of cat flu (herpes- and calicivirus) are classified by the WSAVA as core vaccines, meaning that all cats should receive these vaccines. Herpesvirus often particularly affects the eyes, while calicivirus tends to cause inflammation in the mouth, including ulcers on the tongue.

Cat flu is very common, particularly in the stray population. Most affected animals recover, although some become chronically affected and others, who seemingly recover completely, may become healthy carriers, and remain a source of infection to other cats.

The WSAVA recommends that cats with a high-risk lifestyle receive annual vaccination against herpes- and calicivirus, while cats with a low-risk lifestyle benefit from reducing this to every three years.

Although live vaccines are generally protective after a single dose (as is the case for feline panleukopenia, the other core vaccine for cats), the 2015 version of the WSAVA guidelines points out that some cats seem to require two doses of one of the two cat flu components to mount an antibody response, even when the first one is given after the age of 16 weeks when maternal antibodies no longer play a role. Therefore, at the time of writing, the WSAVA recommends that all cats initially receive two vaccinations against cat flu, regardless of age.

Note that this differs from the situation for dogs.

Leukaemia: non-core killed vaccine

It was the rare but potentially deadly side effects of leukaemia vaccination that first alerted the veterinary community to the need to limit the use of vaccinations. Experts are still not clear on the optimal and/or safest way to use this vaccine. There seems to be a consensus that, if used at all, it should be given to kittens, whereas there is little available evidence to justify its repeated use in adult cats.

Suffice to say that the WSAVA has classified this as a non-core vaccine and, on that basis, I advise against its use in most cases, until further research regarding the effect and safety of the vaccine becomes available.

Please never give the leukaemia vaccine to indoor cats.

Chlamydia: non-core live vaccine

Chlamydia vaccination may be relevant in a cat shelter situation, which is outside the scope of this book. It is not generally recommended for pet cats.

Rabies: killed vaccine

Use of rabies vaccination depends on your geographical region (see page 54). Rabies vaccination is non-core in Australia, New Zealand and much of Europe, where it is relevant only for animals travelling abroad.

If your cat needs a rabies vaccine, make sure to give it at a different time than any other vaccines to minimise the risk of side effects. (See more about rabies on page 53.)

RECOMMENDED VACCINATION PROGRAMME FOR CATS

The kitten series

(1) The three core vaccines – panleukopenia, herpesvirus and calicivirus – are given twice, at 12 and 16 weeks of age (or three times, at ages eight, 12 and 16 weeks).

In some situations where kittens are considered to be at particularly high risk, there may be a benefit in starting the series earlier. If so, three vaccines will be needed, given at eight, 12 and 16 weeks of age.

Checking that the kitten series worked
(2) At five to six months (at least four weeks after the last kitten vaccine), titre test for panleukopenia. This vaccine is known to provide lasting protection, and may protect your cat for his entire life. Once there is a positive titre confirming that the kitten vaccination has provided protection, don't repeat the panleukopenia vaccine without first doing a titre test.

The years ahead
(3) Depending on your cat's lifestyle, you may choose to repeat the cat flu vaccines (herpes- and calicivirus) annually (for cats with outdoor access in areas where they interact with other cats), or less frequently. The WSAVA suggests repeating the cat flu vaccine every three years for cats with a low-risk lifestyle. Make sure that panleukopenia is not needlessly included in this vaccination.

A titre test for panleukopenia every three years or so may be a good idea.

Other vaccines
If you live in an area where rabies vaccination is legally required, or if your cat accompanies you on travels abroad, he needs vaccination against rabies.

Other vaccines are not recommended for routine use. Read more under leukaemia and rabies in this chapter.

Parasites

WORMS, FLEAS AND TICKS

There are not enough pages in this book for me to describe in detail the ideal approach to parasite control for all individual dogs and cats living throughout the world. Instead, I aim in this chapter to discuss our approach to parasite control in general terms.

Irrespective of the obviously large geographical and cultural differences, I want to stress that we all need to urgently rethink how we can best protect our pets from parasites. I believe that we must move away from systematically over-loading both our animals' bodies and our environment with unnecessary chemicals, and instead move toward a much more targeted use of antiparasitic drugs. Regular testing for parasites is one example of how this can be achieved.

In more specific terms, I am going to focus on worms (both intestinal roundworms and French heartworm), fleas and ticks.

Parasites find the weakened and susceptible individual

Our pets may be afflicted by a range of parasites, such as fleas, lice, mites, ticks, and worms. A healthy animal with strong natural resistance will be less susceptible than a weakened individual. If the infection pressure is high enough, even the healthiest animal may succumb to parasitic infection, but, generally speaking, parasitic infection is primarily a problem for young animals and those who are already weakened by other factors, such as disease, medication or poor nutrition.

You could say that for adult animals parasitic problems may, to a certain extent, be the result of an inherent lack of resistance. This holds true for some parasites more than others, and it must be remembered that animals are exposed to very different parasitic burdens, as climates and living conditions vary in different parts of the world.

However, for the majority of healthy adult dogs and cats, parasite prevention does

A healthy resistance

Resistance comes, at least partly, from being in good health. Having healthy genes and leading a healthy lifestyle based on a healthy species-appropriate diet, and a minimum of medicines and toxins provides the strongest immune system and the healthiest gut flora. Remember that resistance is not primarily a consequence of antiparasitic drugs.

not generally require much attention. I would even go so far as to say that this is an area where systematic over-treatment is particularly common, and this is not only detrimental to our pets, but also has far-reaching consequences for the environment.

In northern and western Europe – the areas that I am intimately familiar with as a vet – intestinal worms and fleas are banal infections, which, while requiring treatment if they occur, do not warrant the barrage of

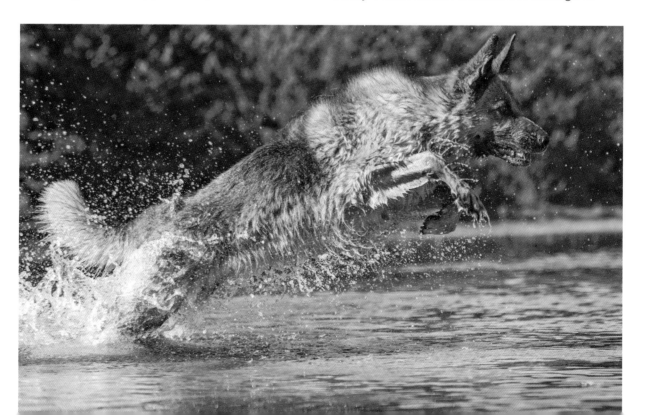

chemicals we still employ simply to prevent these fairly harmless parasites. Heartworms and ticks, on the other hand, potentially pose more serious challenges.

Actually, prevention may *not* be better than cure

People, like pets, may be infected with parasites. Still, we don't, for instance, tend to give our kids a regular worming pill just in case they have become infected with worms since last month. What we do instead is treat for worms (or head lice) when infections occur, as they invariably do at some point with most children. We keep an eye out, we monitor, and only if we find signs of parasitic infections do we treat.

This is a truly sensible approach that I recommend we aim to apply to our animals as well. Bear in mind that the current common practice in many countries of giving regular preventative antiparasitic treatments to dogs and cats in order to prevent them from ever getting fleas or worms is driven primarily by a pharmaceutical industry keen to create a demand. When did you last take a preventative worming pill 'just in case'?

Consider the consequences

The potential for harmful side effects from long-term exposure to absorbed insecticides affecting the health of our dogs and cats is not the only concern. It is simply not a sustainable option to continuously medicate all pet dogs and cats with toxic compounds. If you have the stomach for it, I suggest you Google the effect of neonicotinoid insecticides on the environment. These products are directly linked to the widespread killing of bees and other insects. Imidacloprid is one such neonicotinoid drug, and is the active ingredient in more than 60 different products that we routinely use on our pets (merely to prevent them from getting fleas!). The EU has agreed to ban the agricultural use of neonicotinoid

drugs beginning in 2019; surely, scrutiny of environmental contamination from pet products must be next?

I suggest that we stop using these products irresponsibly today rather than wait for legislation to come into place. As I write this, toxic levels of imidacloprid in UK rivers are already being linked directly to contamination caused by dogs swimming in the water and excreting the drugs in their stool and urine. As well as killing insects who live near streams, these chemicals damage the health of fish and birds, and threaten the life of streams and rivers. It is believed that, in some areas, the use of flea products on dogs is the main cause of environmental contamination, even greater than that caused by the agricultural use of these insecticides.

Test first

Please, keep in mind the overriding principle of testing for parasites, and reserve treatment for when there is an actual harmful parasitic infection. Let us protect our animals and the environment from the constantly repeated blanket treatments.

WORMS

Intestinal worms can be divided into two main groups: roundworms and tapeworms. Adult animals are not normally very affected by these parasites and generally develop a degree of natural resistance.

INTESTINAL ROUNDWORMS (TOXOCARA CANIS AND TOXOCARA CATI)

Puppies and kittens almost always have worms, the explanation for which lies in the incredible lifecycle of the common roundworm: the most common and widespread parasitic worm affecting dogs and cats, and one of the few present around the world. We may call it the 'common' roundworm, but its lifecycle is amazingly complex.

As the young puppy's or kitten's immune system matures, roundworm larvae migrate away from the gut, across the intestinal wall and into the body of the animal, where they settle inside muscle tissue in little curled-up cysts. Inside these cysts, they become completely inactive, and can lie dormant like this, passively hidden away in the muscle tissue, for many years, completely unaffected by worming treatments.

If the animal's immune system later becomes suppressed, perhaps because of illness or medication – or in the case of a female dog, when she becomes pregnant – the parasites 'wake up.' They have, in fact, been lying dormant, waiting for exactly this to happen. Once activated, the worms migrate partly back to the intestines and partly (and how amazing is this) to the placenta and the breast tissue. From here, they infect the new puppies in the womb before they are even born, and continue to do so as whole live worms pass through the milk for many weeks after the puppies are born.

In cats, the same process occurs, with the possible exception that roundworm infection is not believed to happen through the placenta while the kittens are in the womb. Like puppies, however, kittens do become infected with larvae transmitted directly through the milk. This is why we can say for certain that, before they are even old enough to open their eyes or climb out of the nesting box and begin eating solids, puppies and kittens will have been exposed to worms.

Dog and cat roundworms: a human health risk
We have no doubt all seen unhealthy pot-bellied puppies or kittens, and most of us are aware that puppies and kittens should be wormed. While it is certainly true that a heavy worm burden can have a negative impact on the health of young animals, these worms are easily treated, and therefore generally don't cause severe health problems for our pets.

The main reason for focusing on this issue – the real reason, in fact, that this matters so much – is that Toxocara, the common roundworm, while generally not posing a serious health risk to its main hosts (our dogs and cats), can cause very serious illness in humans. This is an example of what is known as a zoonosis: a disease that humans can catch from animals.

Humans are not the intended hosts for this parasite, and the worms cannot mature or multiply in our gut. Instead, when a person (or another accidental host, such as a cow, chicken or sheep) is infected by ingesting eggs shed by a dog, what can happen, probably due to the inbuilt tendency of this parasite to leave the intestinal tract and wander into other tissues as they do in dogs and cats, is a phenomenon called 'larva migrans. 'The worms migrate throughout a person's body, often going completely undetected, but in some cases causing severe injury to the tissues they encounter: typically the liver, lungs, brain or eyes. This is by no means a common syndrome, but it is believed to be severely under-diagnosed, and it is very difficult to treat.

The only way to control this human health problem is to educate pet owners. Once you have seen photos of an eye that has been surgically removed from a young child because it was filled with writhing, live worms, believe me, the image sticks.

This is why we pick up after our dogs.

Now wash your hands
Humans become infected by ingesting worm eggs from soil contaminated with dog excrement. Typically, patients diagnosed with larva migrans are preschool children (most patients are between two and four years old)

who are infected by playing in or even eating dirt. People of all ages are at risk of ingesting toxocara eggs from unwashed hands, or from eating raw, unwashed vegetables. Interestingly, eating uncooked meat from other accidental hosts infected with cysts of toxocara worms, such as chicken or beef, is the major source of human larva migrans in Japan.

Owning a dog is, perhaps surprisingly, not considered a risk factor for people falling ill with larva migrans. This is because the eggs need to mature in the soil for several weeks after being passed by a dog before they become infectious. Contamination, therefore, occurs from soil and not directly from animals.

The eggs of the common roundworm are extremely resilient, and remain infective after lying in the soil for several months; possibly even years. Earthworms, small mammals and birds, as well as rain and wind, further contribute to the spreading of toxocara eggs in the environment. The result is that these eggs are widely present in the soil, even in places like public playgrounds, where fences keep out dogs for precisely this reason.

Larva migrans

Larva migrans (also called toxocariasis) is a public human health concern, and the reason why responsible pet ownership involves diligently worming or testing pregnant and lactating bitches, as well as puppies under six months. It is also why it is so important to always pick up after our dogs

The rational use of intestinal worming treatments

Roundworms are only rarely excreted by healthy adult animals. In fact, intestinal worms seldom cause adult dogs and cats any health problems. It follows, then, that regular worming of adult cats and dogs against intestinal worms is neither logical nor defensible. By all means, if your adult dog or cat vomits up worms or you see worms in their stool, give them a wormer. In the absence of these clear signs, they are highly unlikely to benefit from worming.

Worms are excreted almost exclusively by pregnant and lactating bitches and queens, and by young puppies and kittens. For the sake of animal and human health alike, it is crucial that breeders don't neglect to worm the bitch during pregnancy, and repeat worming treatments several times for both the puppies and their mother during the first eight weeks of life. If the breeder decides against routine worming, repeated faecal testing is absolutely vital. Thorough worming while the roundworms are still in the gut, where they can be reached by wormers, will reduce the number of worms that migrate into the dog's tissues, and thereby limit the egg excretion for the rest of his life.

The young puppies should therefore continue to be regularly wormed until they are six months old. Once they are past puberty, however, regular worming for roundworms is a waste of time and, from the point of view of intestinal worms at least, the worming of adults (apart from pregnant or lactating females) should be reduced to those showing clear signs of parasitic infection.

Bum scooting or licking is generally not associated with worms in dogs and cats the way itchy bums are in children. In dogs, exaggerated interest in their rear end is much more likely to be due to other causes, such as discomfort stemming from the anal glands.

Adult animals tend to develop a natural resistance against intestinal worms, and if they do get a bad case, they'll show signs of this and you can worm them, in keeping with the way worms are treated when they occur in humans. Nothing is gained from regular indiscriminate worming for intestinal worms, except a pointless toxic burden that affects both the individual animal and the environment. Apart from the mothers and offspring described above, there is simply no risk-based argument to defend routine worming in dogs and cats. Instead, just treat them if they do get worms.

A safe alternative?

Increasingly, conscientious breeders choose to abandon blanket preventative worm treatments in favour of worm testing. In light of the lifecycle of the common roundworm, it is interesting that not all puppies and pregnant bitches test positive when their stool is examined for toxocara eggs.

One explanation for this could be that the bitch was so thoroughly wormed as a pup that she has only negligible stores of dormant larvae. If you veer from the recommendation of routine worming against Toxocara canis in puppies and their mothers, it is imperative, for the sake of the dogs as well as for reasons of public health, to get repeated stool samples examined.

The who's who of heart- and lungworm in dogs

Angiostrongylus vasorum (French heartworm) is discussed in the main text. This is the one we worry about in Europe.
Crenosoma vulpis (fox's lungworm) has a similar lifecycle but causes much milder, if any, symptoms, and is never fatal to dogs.
Oslerus osleri (dog's lungworm) is spread directly through dog faeces. It is found worldwide, but is mostly problematic in kennel conditions.
Dirofilaria immitis (tropical heartworm) is a tropical disease: infection is spread by mosquitoes.

ANGIOSTRONGYLUS VASORUM (FRENCH HEARTWORM)

Angiostrongylus vasorum is also called French heartworm, and sometimes referred to as lungworm. This parasite is passed on to dogs via snails and slugs, and, to a lesser degree, frogs. The dog picks up larvae by swallowing, licking or even just sniffing the slug, snail or the trails they leave behind. The larvae then go through the dog's liver and migrate through the body, ending up as adult worms in the pulmonary artery or the right side of the heart. Here, they lay eggs, which hatch into new larvae and move to the lungs, where they are coughed up, swallowed, and passed in the stool. The larvae are then picked up by slugs or snails, and the whole slimy cycle starts again.

Please note that dogs don't have to do any more than drink from a puddle or an outside water bowl, eat some grass or play with a ball or a stick that has been lying outside. Think of the shiny trails that you see everywhere on a misty summer morning. Also note that dogs don't pass this infection on to each other or, indeed, to humans. This is why it is very common for one dog to become infected (often repeatedly) with French heartworm while other dogs in the same household never do. It is the dog with the high-risk behaviour (such as eating everything) who will typically become infected, and often re-infected, while many other dogs in the same local environment remain uninfected.

Snails and larvae both do best in warm and humid conditions, and the risk of infection is highest in spring and summer when snails are most active. Vets who practice in areas where French heartworm infection is common will know that dogs are typically brought to the vet with symptoms of disease in the autumn. This is because it generally takes several months from the time infection is picked up (in spring and summer) until the dog begins to show signs of becoming ill.

Symptoms of French heartworm infection

The most common symptoms of French

heartworm infection are coughing and lack of energy. In other (more serious) cases, the primary symptoms are bleeding irregularities, which are often noticed as redness (bleeding) in the gums or the whites of the eyes.

Fox lungworm (Crenosoma vulpis) also infects dogs, and is generally more common than French heartworm. The symptoms of infection are quite mild and rarely present a serious health threat. This parasite is mainly worth knowing about because it has a similar lifecycle to, and can easily be mistaken for, French heartworm (angiostrongylus vasorum).

In areas where these parasites exist, your vet will naturally test for heart- and lungworm infection if your dog shows any of these symptoms. The point of regular testing is to catch infection before it causes your dog any discomfort – we want early detection to ensure that we can treat the infection before the parasite has a chance to cause disease.

Who gets French heartworm?

The main factors that influence your dog's risk of becoming infected are the region where you live, the time of year, his behaviour and, finally, his age. French heartworm is only present in certain geographical regions, and within those areas, only during certain times of the year.

An unusual characteristic of this parasite is that it may be common in one area while, just a hundred kilometres away, it may be rare or non-existent. Find out if you are living in a French heartworm hotspot: your local veterinarians should know. If you are living in an area with a high incidence of French heartworm, be aware that in countries where the winter temperature regularly goes below freezing, this is a seasonal problem that you don't have to worry about in the winter months. Infections will happen during the spring and summer and typically cause problems in late summer and autumn.

Finally, this is predominantly a problem that affects young dogs who have immature immune systems, and tend to be the ones who eat everything, so are therefore much more likely to ingest snails. Most cases are seen in dogs who are less than 18 months old, and very few are seen in dogs over two years of age. Furthermore, those who do become infected at a greater age have generally had the infection before, simply because the dog in question is likely to be of the curious, all-devouring type.

In summary, this means that, in the middle of winter, outside of a geographical hotspot, or if your dog is an adult who has never had a French heartworm infection before, the risk of infection is negligible. It is difficult to see the rationale for regularly worming dogs of all ages, in all areas, all year round, as some TV commercials would suggest we should.

Risk factors

The two main risk factors for French heartworm (angiostrongylus) infection are:
Geographical area (some areas have no French heartworm while others are known hotspots of infection)
Age of your dog (the vast majority of cases are in dogs less than 18 months old)

What can you do about the risk of heart- and lungworm infection?

First of all, don't panic. If you have seen the TV advertising campaigns advocating regular heart- and lungworm prevention, stop for a second and consider who made those ads. They are, indeed, not public service announcements for the advancement of dog health; rather, they are commercials produced by pharmaceutical companies that want to sell a product, and are not embarrassed to use fear as a marketing tool.

Second, let's look at what can be done to minimise the risk of infection. Remember those misty morning snail trails from earlier? We want to prevent these getting into your dog's mouth. Whilst you can never eliminate this contact, it is certainly possible to greatly reduce it by taking a few common sense steps.

As far as possible, prevent your dog from drinking out of puddles (if you have a thirsty dog, get into the habit of taking water with you on walks), and from eating grass. Don't have an outdoor water bowl or leave dog toys outside overnight. If your dog enjoys garden time with a favourite bone or ball, pick up the toys at the end of the day and take them indoors overnight. Spreading a handful of dry dog food or treats on the ground outside is great occupational therapy and nose work, but it is not a good idea from the point of view of parasite prevention. I strongly recommend that you don't do this. On the contrary, aim to teach your dog to not eat from the ground.

There are many other sniffing games that can take the place of searching for food tidbits. You can just as easily hide a toy or even a treat in a bowl before you let your dog outside, or you can feed his food or treats in a toy designed to make him work to get at it. All I am saying is please don't spread food directly on the ground or lawn.

Another useful measure to reduce the spread of infection of all kinds is to always pick up and properly dispose of dog poo.

Herbal supplements, garlic, diatomaceous earth, and other products often marketed as alternatives to conventional wormers are not effective against heart- and lungworm infection. The lifecycle of these parasites means that they are only present in the intestinal canal for a very short time.

Third, in place of routinely giving conventional worming treatments, I recommend using regular testing for at-risk dogs in order to pick up signs of infection. This can be done though a blood test, but it is often easier and cheaper to have a stool sample examined for larvae. You can hand in a stool sample to your vet, who may examine it herself or send it on to a lab, or you can send it straight to the lab yourself (see page 216).

How to collect a stool sample

You want a fresh and clean sample that hasn't touched the ground. While it may be possible to catch the stool in a bag mid-air or as it leaves your dog, often, the more realistic option is to pinch off a piece from the top of a fresh stool. You only need an amount equivalent to a teaspoonful. Collect a sample on three consecutive days and drop off the three bags together at your vet's, or send them directly to a laboratory offering this service.

When testing for French heartworm, it is counterproductive to keep the stool samples cool. Room temperature is ideal, which means that you may have to keep the samples indoors during winter.

Test before you treat

Proactive parasite control as an alternative to regular preventative worming: get your dog's stool tested at regular intervals to ensure that any worms present will be discovered before they have a chance to cause symptoms and do harm. This way, your dog is only exposed to antiparasitic chemicals if he needs them. A suggested protocol for those living in areas affected by French heartworm would be to send off stool samples from young dogs (under two years old) and previously infected dogs of any age every two months between early spring and the onset of winter.

If your dog has heart- or lungworm

If your dog is diagnosed with French heartworm or lungworm, he must, of course, be treated by your vet with one of the available antiparasitic drugs. With a timely diagnosis, the treatment is, in most cases, easy and effective, and dogs respond well to early treatment.

Early detection is the key to preventing deaths or irreversible damage to the heart and lungs. Infected dogs often suffer recurrences, not because the treatment failed to work, but because the behaviour that led to the first infection continues. For this reason, if your dog has once had an infection and has been treated for it, it is crucial to continue checking with extra vigilance, even after he has checked clear once or twice. Hand in the stool samples to your vet or send them directly to a lab yourself every two months during the relevant season.

Cat lungworm (Aelurostrongylus abstrusus)

As just described for Angiostrongylus in dogs, snails are also the intermediate host for cat lungworm, meaning that the larvae undergo a necessary stage of their development in snails (so infection cannot exist without snails).

However, it is believed that cats are primarily infected not through snails but rather through eating birds and mice that in turn ate the snails. It follows that only cats with outdoor access, and an interest and skill in hunting are at risk.

The symptoms are respiratory problems such as coughing, wheezing, sneezing and nasal discharge. Some infected cats show no symptoms. The diagnosis is made by examining stool samples for larvae. The vet may examine the sample herself or send it off to a lab, or you may send it directly to a lab yourself.

FLEAS

Ctenocephalides cati, the cat flea, is the most common flea to infest our animals. The cat flea thrives on both cat and dog blood. It may even enjoy the occasional sip of human blood, although it cannot sustain itself or multiply on a human blood meal.

Does your home have fleas?

Once the first flea has found its way into your home on the back of a dog or cat, it is no longer a matter of each animal having fleas. Rather, once your home has been infected and the first eggs are present in the cracks and corners of your home, it is the house that has fleas. Sure, one cat in the household may scratch incessantly while another does not scratch at all. There is huge variation in how fleabites affect each dog or cat. Animals who are allergic to flea saliva will scratch much more and for much longer from each bite, but that does not mean that one cat has fleas while another doesn't; it simply means that one is more sensitive to the fleabites. Once one of your animals has brought home one flea, your home has fleas. It's that simple.

The life of a flea

The adult flea spends a significant part of its life hidden away on the host animal, in this case your dog or cat, where it consumes a blood meal, mates, and lays eggs. The eggs, however, don't stay on the dog's or cat's body, but are deposited in the surroundings, and end up spread all around your home, where they subsequently hatch in every nook and cranny. A single female flea can lay several hundred eggs, which go on to hatch in your carpets, rugs, sofas, beds, and between your floorboards.

The eggs hatch after about a week, and out come larvae, which continue to move around your home, venturing further into gaps and cracks before they pupate. The pupal stage can last from a few days to many months before the pupa hatches, and a new flea emerges ready to look for a host animal (dog or cat) to provide the blood meal needed for it to lay eggs and continue the cycle.

Once a flea infestation has taken hold, only about 1% of the flea population in your home will consist of adult fleas. The remaining 99% is made up of eggs, larvae and pupae. These 'invisible' juvenile stages are not on your dog or cat but rather spread around your home. This is why it is truly the house that has fleas and not the individual animal, and why flea treatment has to take this into account.

Spot the flea

A flea infestation is only rarely discovered by someone happening to spot a flea. Suspicion is generally raised because of a dramatic increase in a dog's or cat's scratching and grooming behaviour. If you should see one or more fleas on your animal, you can safely assume that the infestation in your home has already reached significant proportions: that one flea is truly the tip of the iceberg.

On the other hand, you can easily have a house full of fleas without being able to spot a single flea on your dog – and seeing fleas on cats is even less likely. You will only rarely spot live adult fleas on your dog and almost never on your cat. The juvenile stages of a flea are too small to see with the naked

eye. Thus, while you may discover that you have a flea problem by spotting a flea, this is unlikely. Much more commonly, you'll notice an increase in your animal's scratching behaviour. Some people, myself included, are so sensitive to fleabites that the tell-tale itchy red spots on our lower legs serve as red flags, alerting us to the presence of fleas.

It is said that fleas hide so successfully in thick cat fur, and that cats clean themselves so fastidiously, that you stand a better chance of finding an ingested flea in a cat stool sample than seeing it on your cat. If there are lots of fleas around, you may spot one or two on your dog if you look for them. Fleas move fast, and avoid exposure to light. To increase your chance of spotting fleas on your dog, find a well-lit place and roll him over so that his lower belly and armpits are suddenly exposed to light. You may then catch a brief glimpse of the tiny black beasts darting for cover. After only a second, they will be gone, hidden again in the furry depths ...

The comb check is, perhaps, a more reliable way to actively check for fleas. It doesn't show you fleas, but it will reliably show you the next best thing as sure proof of their presence: flea excrement, often called flea dirt.

Run a fine-toothed comb through the coat at the end of the back near the base of the tail a couple of times, then tap the comb on a dampened piece of white kitchen towel. Any dust or other debris that remains black is nothing to worry about, but if the black specks

Flea spotting

Fleas are notoriously difficult to see. When you do spot them, it will be by suddenly exposing them in areas without much fur. Turn over your dog in a well-lit place and look for movement around his groin and armpits. Be prepared as you will barely have a second before they are gone. You'll know it when you see one.

from the comb dissolve into reddish-brown streaks or blotches upon contact with the wet paper, they are, in fact, flea excrement. The reddish colour comes from the high content of blood within the flea dirt, and is a sure sign that your house has fleas.

Preventing fleas

While fleas are common parasites, they are not dangerous; nor do they carry any serious diseases. I therefore see little justification for applying toxic chemicals in order to prevent fleas. What is the worst that can happen from omitting preventative flea treatments? Well, you could get fleas – and then it would make sense to treat for them. In fact, if we reserve chemicals against fleas to the situations where a flea infestation has actually happened, we would no doubt have fewer problems with fleas developing resistance to the drugs, and we would, of course, dramatically reduce the exposure of our pets to these known toxic substances, as well as reduce environmental contamination.

One thing is certain: once fleas have been introduced (that is, once your house has fleas), there is no benefit from any treatment aimed at deterring fleas. That ship has sailed. If your animals are scratching, if you have found flea dirt using the comb check, or if you have seen as much as a single flea on your animal, your house has already well and truly got fleas. You can forget about prevention and move straight to eradication. If there is one flea, there will be thousands, and the eggs and other juvenile stages will already be everywhere.

Eradicating fleas

It doesn't really make sense to talk about flea infestations as a matter of degree. Some people are under the impression that a dog or cat may be unfortunate enough to suffer a bite from the occasional passing flea. This is not the case. You either have fleas or you don't.

It is not (at least not for very long) a question of how many fleas you have, or a matter of reducing the number of fleas. Having fleas is an all or nothing situation.

You may well have a dog or cat for a decade – indeed, for their entire lifetime – without ever getting fleas, but once you have them, in the absence of treatment, they will never go away without a sustained and targeted effort, as described below.

Flea combing makes little sense. You may catch one or two out of hundreds or probably thousands, and you will never be able to make an impact on the huge supply of eggs and larvae waiting to mature. You will never see these juvenile stages, as they are too small for the naked eye. Nor will any amount of cleaning have any real impact, since they are all nicely hidden away in dark, unreachable corners, and the eggs have a sticky surface that means they will not be removed by hoovering.

So, you have two options. You can focus only on treating your cats and dogs, or you can include spraying the house to target the juvenile stages as well. If you choose the former approach, the key is to keep up the treatment until there isn't a single unhatched egg or pupa in the house, which will take at least six months, and maybe even longer in unheated rooms.

A very common scenario goes like this. You discover that you have fleas, and you begin treating the animals in the house. You quickly notice an improvement as your animals scratch less. After two or three months, the scratching has ceased, and you haven't spotted any fleas for a long time. It seems that the fleas have gone, and you cease the treatments.

Skip ahead a few months and it seems that you have picked up fleas again as the manic scratching resumes. What has really happened, however, is that the treatment reduced the flea burden for a while, but as

Getting the needle

I very much enjoyed the response of a renowned veterinary herbalist and acupuncturist, when she was asked at a seminar how she would use holistic methods to treat flea infestations. Her answer was that, in her experience, acupuncture needles worked better than herbs – but you do need to have really quick reflexes ...

soon as the treatment stopped, allowing newly-hatched fleas to feed and lay eggs, the population increased again. You didn't catch fleas again; you had fleas all along, and have them still. The level of the on-going infestation increased just enough to make them noticeable again.

The key is to keep up the treatment with no gaps so that no new eggs can be laid until the available pool of eggs and pupae have all hatched. While improvement will be noticeable soon after you start treatment, the fleas will invariably return unless you keep up the treatment until there isn't a single viable egg left in the house.

There are a multitude of insecticides available for use on dogs and cats. None of them is pleasant to use, which is why I recommend reserving them for when there are actually fleas to treat. There have been a number of reported cases of serious (even fatal) side effects attributed to the flea products that are administered in tablet form. Therefore, for the time being, I recommend sticking with well-known products that have been around for a while; especially collars or pour-on products. The pour-on products are still systemically absorbed pesticides, but while I don't use them lightly, the worst obvious side effects I have seen from these products are localised allergic skin reactions.

Unlike when kids get lice ('nits'), it is important to appreciate that the adult fleas present on your dog or cat constitute only a very small part of the problem. The vast majority of fleas are the juvenile stages spread all over your home. It is crucial to bear this in mind when planning your treatment (eradication) strategy. An adult flea needs a blood meal from a dog or cat in order to lay eggs and continue the family line. It is, therefore, possible to eradicate fleas from your home entirely by applying insecticides to your dog and cat.

Methoprene

You will be able to speed up the flea eradication and cease treatment sooner if you combine treating the animals with targeting the juvenile stages in the environment. In this way, you cut off the problem at the root, instead of waiting for each immature flea to mature before the treatment is effective.

Look for a spray containing the active ingredient methoprene. Methoprene is a biological insecticide that interferes with the maturation of the larvae by mimicking a larval growth hormone. It is non-toxic to mammals as well as to pupae or adult fleas.

Spray the whole house, including areas your animals don't have access to, and don't forget to spray your car, and also your office if you take your dog to work.

TICKS

Tick bites, in and of themselves, are rarely a problem, although if a tick should be incompletely removed so that the mouth parts are accidentally left embedded in the skin, this may cause a local irritant reaction.

The reason we are concerned about ticks, however, is not to do with the ticks themselves, but rather because of the risk of serious diseases, such as anaplasmosis and borreliosis (Lyme disease), being transmitted via tick bites.

The longer a tick remains attached, the

higher the risk that it will transfer disease. Regularly check your dog and cat for ticks, and always remove them as soon as you discover them. The risk of disease is considered to be minimal if ticks are removed within a few hours of attaching, so if you live in an area with lots of ticks, get in the habit of checking your dog after each walk in grassy or woody areas.

It's not difficult to incorporate tick checks into your daily schedule. If you teach your dog to be still for a tick check at the end of a walk and reward him for his cooperation, this will quickly become habit for all involved. Removing a tick from a squirming dog, however, is no easy task.

Neither the tick bite itself nor having the tick pulled off hurts at all, and removal is another example of the value of teaching your dog to allow himself to be restrained and handled from an early age (ear inspections, nail clipping, and so on, fall into this category of necessary handling skills). You may need someone to help you keep your dog or cat still so that you can focus on removing the tick, but being able to perform this simple task without help means that you can do it without delay whenever you spot a tick. Early removal is essential, as it greatly reduces the risk of disease transmission.

Yes, ticks are gross and potentially the source of serious disease, but most dog carers become so used to dealing with them in a timely and matter-of-fact fashion that they will discover and swiftly remove a tick from their dog, without even pausing in conversation to do so. There is really nothing to it.

Removing ticks

A tick that is quickly discovered and completely removed poses no great threat. The more ticks your dog has, and the longer they are left in place, the greater the risk.

To remove a tick embedded in the skin of a dog or cat (or human), the trick is to pull it out promptly and cleanly without squeezing or breaking it. Ideally, you should avoid leaving the mouth parts of the tick in the skin as this can cause some irritation, but if this happens, don't worry. Just keep an eye on the area for a few days; most likely it will heal without problems.

The main point when removing a tick is that it should be done in one steady movement.

Carefully separate the hairs around the tick so you can see what you are doing, and get a good grip on the tick itself, and pull it out. You may hear of methods intended to induce the tick to let go. Suffocating it by covering it with petroleum jelly, burning it or making it let go by applying lavender oil, tea tree oil, alcohol or other substances are all examples of such common (but dangerous) myths. Never use these methods. If the tick is stressed into letting go, there is a much greater risk that it will salivate or regurgitate into the bite wound, meaning that, by using these methods, you are actually increasing the risk of disease being transmitted. It is probably safer to leave the tick in place than to repel it by applying anything to it.

Inasfar as ticks are conscious of anything (I'm not going there), you want to remove it quickly and effectively by pulling it out before it knows what is happening. There are plenty of tools available for the swift, easy and complete removal of ticks. If you don't have one on you when you discover a tick on your dog or cat, a pair of pointed tweezers works just as well. If you don't have immediate access to tweezers or other tick removers, you can also use your fingers. The advantage of tweezers and tick removers is that they enable you to grab hold of the tick very close to where it is attached to the skin so you avoid grabbing its body.

Using your fingers is better than leaving the tick attached for several hours longer. When you remove a tick with your fingers, you have no choice but to hold onto its body. Don't squeeze the tick's body; rather, hold it gently and pull in a steady motion. I must admit I find it easier to hold the body between two fingers and turn clockwise (at the wrist, not by twirling the tick), though the general recommendation is to pull it straight out rather than turning it.

Whatever works for you: just don't squeeze and don't jerk – and don't worry.

A lint roller or similar adhesive tool designed for removing animal hairs from clothing and furniture is an excellent way to remove crawling ticks from the fur of a large hairy dog immediately after a walk. This method won't catch ticks that have already managed to attach themselves, but it can remove even the tiniest, almost invisible tick crawling in the dog's fur before it has a chance to attach. This is a great tool if your dog is of a size and coat type that makes complete tick checks challenging.

Tick removal

Never apply anything to a tick in order to make it let go. This only increases the risk of disease transmission. Instead, just pull it out.

What about natural products for parasite control?

I have to confess that I remain sceptical about so-called natural methods of parasite control. I believe that truly natural methods can only achieve a truly natural state, and it is, in fact, not natural to be free of parasites.

The wild ancestors of our pets would certainly have been carrying parasites, but generally the balance would have been such that the parasites would not have seriously compromised the health of their host – killing the host is clearly not in the best interest of any parasite.

Our modern interpretation of cleanliness, and our standard of living mean that we don't accept parasites as an unavoidable part of life, and that our living conditions (installation of central heating and abandoning a nomadic lifestyle) differ greatly from those of earlier times, often shifting the balance in the parasites' favour.

We must limit the use of systemic pesticides ...

I think it is imperative that we make sure to only expose our animals to an absolute minimum of chemicals. If you are not reluctant to give your dogs and cats pesticides, I think it is probably only because you haven't really given it much thought. Whether the antiparasitic drug is absorbed through the skin or given in tablet form, it is absorbed by the animal, the consequence being that their whole body is subjected to what is, by its very nature, an insecticide – not something you would want to take internally.

People are also affected by parasites such as lice and ticks, but I think we would all baulk at the idea of treating ourselves with a systemically-absorbed chemical that killed these beasts on contact with our skin, and no doubt we would be even more reluctant to repeat such treatments regularly throughout our entire lives. Nevertheless, many conscientious dog and cat owners do this, often on their vet's advice, and always with the best intentions – but sometimes with very little justification.

... but simply substituting them with other products may not be the answer

Make no mistake; I am very reluctant to use systemic pesticides, or to recommend their use for my patients. Having said that, I am not sure that the best answer is simply to substitute one product (the conventional antiparasitic drugs recommended by your vet) for a so-called alternative or natural version.

There are many such products available, with more popping up every day.

The recommendations are many, and the alternative pet product market is booming. Common recommendations include garlic and brewer's yeast to deter just about anything; diatomaceous earth given both internally and distributed in the environment as a treatment for both worms and fleas, not to mention a plethora of products based on the insect-deterrent properties of strong smells: neem oil, tea tree oil, and other essential oils (aromatherapy oils), such as lavender, citronella and lemongrass form the basis of many products that are applied to discourage fleas and ticks.

On the one hand, I think that the use of essential oils to deter ticks is probably the natural antiparasitic approach that makes the most sense. I can certainly imagine that a strong smell could prevent ticks from searching out an individual. On the other hand, the thought of applying a product to dogs, whose sense of smell is so keen, intended to work by giving off strong odours, concerns me. I imagine that walking around doused in aromatic essences must be a constant stress factor for a dog, akin to the sensory overload experienced by a person suffering from tinnitus. Besides, as a homeopath, I am constantly advising against the use of garlic, essential oils (aromatherapy), and other strong-smelling substances, as they interfere with the effect of homeopathic medicines.

More often than not, it is not a matter of these products being harmful; rather, their use is undocumented in dogs and cats, and most of all, they are not needed. At the very least, let us use all products with caution, and remember that whether 'conventional' or 'alternative,' all these products have the potential to cause harm – and should be used with care.

'Natural' does not necessarily mean safe

I have never really been a fan of 'products,' and I have never sold anything but information.

A practical approach

There is no totally safe and effective product for use against parasites. Beware of those that claim otherwise, whether they are keen to sell you conventional antiparasitic drugs based on active ingredients such as imidacloprid or fipronil, or so-called alternative treatments like lavender oil, garlic or diatomaceous earth. I recommend a common sense approach, relying on awareness of the real risk in the local environment, and utilising testing in lieu of blanket routine treatments.

I appreciate that many feel differently, and that the idea of finding a panacea, or of simply buying something nice for one's dog or cat, appeals to many. I am absolutely not trying to imply that none of the available products or supplements have a role to play; only to recommend that they are used with critical thought and an awareness of the fact that just because something is 'natural,' does not mean it is inherently safe or innocuous.

Some of the commonly recommended and used substances (neem oil, tea tree oil, diatomaceous earth) can be irritants to the airways, sometimes causing severe reactions. Many natural products can cause allergic reactions when applied to the skin. As described in the chapter on diet (see page 30), garlic should be used with caution in dogs as it can damage their red blood cells, resulting in haemolytic anaemia. Most dogs can no doubt tolerate small amounts of fresh garlic without problems, but there is, in my view, really no reason for giving it. How is a dog eating garlic natural anyway? Some dogs are more sensitive to the toxicity of garlic than others, and there is always a risk that the harmful effect may build over time from regular dosing.

My point here is primarily that there are many reasons why we cannot simply extrapolate from humans to animals, and that we should be careful about applying products of any kind when there may be no real need or benefit. Adult dogs and cats certainly don't need alternative wormers. There may be a benefit to alternative tick deterrents if they are safe, don't overwhelm the dog's sensitive sense of smell, and don't have any side effects.

There is no logic to applying products that deter fleas if the animal, or rather the household, already has them.

Herbal tea, kitty?

While I have no objection at all to giving herbal supplements to dogs and cats, I recommend using them in a targeted way when there is a specific rationale behind the treatment (see the chapter on herbal medicine page 103). I suspect, however, that the current trend of including 'mixtures of good herbs' in many foods, treats and supplements for dogs and cats (often without proper labelling of ingredients) is mostly about appealing to consumers. Sometimes, terms like 'natural' and 'beneficial' are defined so vaguely as to make no real sense at all. I think we should critically consider what can reasonably be considered a natural supplement for a carnivore.

Natural wormers

Adult dogs don't generally suffer from intestinal worms, as they tend to build up a natural resistance, and so don't require or benefit from any preventative treatments. Furthermore, as mentioned above, young animals and their mothers need conventional wormers. Omitting such treatment would be highly irresponsible, and constitute a human public health concern.

French heartworm, a more serious issue in some geographical areas, only spend a brief period in the gut before entering the airways, meaning that they cannot be effectively controlled by the presence of substances in the gut, such as herbs or diatomaceous earth. Knowing of dogs who have been infected by French heartworm while supposedly protected by herbal wormers, I am worried about the false sense of security such products may induce in the face of a real parasitic threat. I am also by nature keen on the general principle of keeping things simple, and I do not believe in administering a product or substance (be it a vaccine, a supplement or any medicine) for which there is not sufficient safety information, and, most of all, the benefit of which has not been established.

In most situations, the effective way to reduce the use of pesticides centres around knowing the prevalence of parasites in your area, and understanding their lifecycles so that you can use tests and treatments in a targeted way that limits their use to susceptible individuals in affected areas during the relevant times of year.

In summary – general points on parasite control

I am sorry to tell you that I don't have a magic solution or (I wish!) a product that safely and effectively rids your animal of all parasite problems. I think I am aware of most of the products available and the claims made about them, and I suppose all I can helpfully say is beware of those that claim to have such a solution, be it in the form of conventional or alternative treatments. My advice is to limit the use of antiparasitic products (conventional and alternative), and use regular testing rather than regular preventative treatments. When possible, reserve treatment for the cases where we *know* that parasites are present.

There are too many geographical and climate variations, as well as differences in lifestyle, for me to be able to recommend a certain specific parasite prevention regime, so let me just say this. For the vast majority of dogs and cats, no preventative treatment regime of any kind is needed. If your vet recommends that you give your adult pet a regular treatment to avoid becoming infected with fleas, ticks or worms, I suggest you pause, think, and look into the necessity of such treatments. Establish what the risks are in your area, and whether it is possible to monitor the situation through regular targeted testing rather than blindly treating.

As discussed above, fleas and intestinal worms in adult dogs rarely warrant attention unless you see signs of parasitic infections. Save your animal and the environment from unnecessary chemical exposure, and aim instead to deal with the parasitic problem if it actually occurs.

In the case of other worms and of ticks, you will have to use your judgement. Remember, the overriding principle of good medicine is to only give a medicine that is actually required.

In summary – main points and recommendations about specific parasites

Worms

•   Intestinal worms

Diligently worm or test lactating bitches and puppies until the age of six months. This is for their protection, but just as importantly it is your duty, as this is a human public health issue. After that age, don't worry unless there are signs of worms.

The same recommendation applies to lactating queens and kittens. Cats who hunt outdoors may catch worms from their prey. Treat if you see signs of worms only. In most situations, there is no justification or need for any preventative worming treatments or supplements against intestinal worms in adult dogs or cats.

Once they are adults, you can forget about it unless you see worms, and only then should you treat.

•   French heartworm

This parasite can cause serious health problems, but cannot spread directly between dogs. Because a dog can only become infected via snails and slugs, the parasite affects only certain geographical areas at certain times of year, and then only dogs displaying certain behaviours. Find out about the prevalence in your area. In many areas, no measures are needed at all. Even if you live in a French heartworm (angiostrongylus) hotspot and have a middle-aged dog who has never been affected, it is overwhelmingly likely that he is not displaying high-risk behaviour, and is therefore not at a level of risk that justifies ongoing preventative wormers.

Instead, you may wish to test his stools a few times, and take common sense precautions (don't throw treats on the ground or leave toys outside overnight, and so on). If you live in an area affected by French heartworm and you have a dog under the age of 18 months, or a dog of any age who has previously been treated for a diagnosed French heartworm infection, I recommend testing every other month from spring till late autumn. I cannot support regular preventative treatments.

Fleas

You may choose to use a constant deterrent in an attempt to avoid bringing home that first flea. However, this involves a lot of treatments over an animal's lifetime to avoid something that is not even a health threat, and has no serious consequences should it occur. There are also the issues of environmental contamination and of parasites developing resistance to treatments. While there are many alternative deterrent methods, be aware that they may carry risks, too.

Once fleas have been introduced into your home, taking steps to deter them or reduce their number makes little sense. Eradication must involve all dogs and cats in the house, and must be carried out for a sufficiently long period of time (many months).

If you simply stop as soon as there are no more signs of fleas, the infestation will regrow from remaining pupae.

Ticks

Ticks only concern us because of the potential for disease transmission through tick bites. There is no reason for you to consider tick prevention if your dog or cat has a lifestyle, or lives in an area, that means he simply doesn't get ticks.

The most important step to prevent transmission of tick-borne diseases is to inspect your animal daily and remove ticks correctly and immediately when you discover them.

However, if your animal gets a large number of ticks, you'll need to consider anti-tick treatments. There are a number of products available on the market. I recommend that you limit their use to situations where the risks of the pesticide are clearly outweighed by the risk of the tick-borne disease. You may be able to reduce the number of ticks on your dog simply by keeping him away from forested areas and long grass. You may also find safe and nontoxic sprays that you can apply before each walk to deter ticks. If your dog keeps getting several ticks every week, and you are unable to find and remove them immediately, the safest option is to use a veterinary pesticide during the tick season. These products have the added bonus of also deterring fleas.

I suggest that you stay away from newly-released products, and that you regard with caution pesticides that are to be taken orally (in tablet or pill form).

Please note that while the information about common roundworms and fleas is globally relevant, other parasite challenges vary depending on geographical area. I refrain, for instance, from offering any advice regarding the treatment of tropical parasites such as the tropical heartworm (Dirofillaria immitis). Always consult your local vet for information about the local risk of parasitic infections.

Read the chapter on page 37 about choosing the right vet, and look for someone who is not simply rehashing the drug company rep's sales pitch, but who has remained critical and educated about the real local risks. The aim is always to reserve treatment for situations in which there is an actual need, so do ask local vets what serious parasitic diseases they actually see in your area.

Always return to the principle of testing rather than preventative treatment whenever possible.

Visit Hubble and Hattie on the web: www.hubbleandhattie.com
hubbleandhattie.blogspot.co.uk
• Details of all books • Special offers • Newsletter • New book news

75

Neutering

SPAYING, CASTRATION, AND ALL THINGS SEXUAL

The procedure of de-sexing or neutering goes under many different names, with castration, sterilisation, altering, fixing, spaying and speying being just a few of these. I will use neutering as a common term referring to the de-sexing of both males (castration), and females (spaying).

Surprising new insights

This topic, more than any other, reflects the large geographical and cultural differences in our approach to keeping dogs. It is also an area where big changes are happening.

In contrast to the situation with dogs, there seems to be worldwide consensus regarding how best to manage cat sexuality. There is perhaps some discussion about the optimal timing of neutering, but, overall, everyone pretty much agrees about cats, and little has changed on that front in recent years.

Not so when it comes to dogs.

It all started with a big study from the University of California, Davis, that was published in 2013. Researchers analysed the lifetime health records of 759 Golden Retrievers, and compared the health of neutered dogs to that of intact dogs. Very

New advice

From around 2017, experts around the world agree that, according to new evidence, it is no longer possible to recommend blanket routine neutering of dogs.

surprisingly, they found a significantly increased risk of both cancer and joint disease in the neutered animals. This sparked a frenzy of research into the effects of neutering, which has now become one of the hottest areas in veterinary research (so continue to watch this space).

From around 2017, experts have certainly agreed that it is no longer possible to recommend blanket routine neutering of dogs. Owners must be informed of the risks involved, and understand that, in some cases, the dog's health may be harmed through neutering.

There now seems to be statistical evidence to show that intact dogs live longer than neutered dogs. This is not related to any one disease or major cause of death in neutered animals, but a general beneficial effect on health of life-long exposure to sexual hormones.

One study from 2016 states, 'It has

Pros and cons

Generally speaking, you could argue that, from an holistic viewpoint, it must be preferable to leave an animal intact, as the hormonal system has a profound influence on the whole body, and is not limited to the area of reproduction. Therefore, intact animals are more natural: healthier, more complete beings. On the other hand, being sexually intact but denied the opportunity to act on the hormonal impulse to reproduce is (for animals at least) far from a natural situation. The answer has to be a careful weighing of pros and cons. Luckily, research in recent years has shed new light on the consequences that neutering has on behaviour, physical health and longevity, helping us to make informed decisions.

become clear that canine gonads (sexual organs, ie: ovaries and testicles) are not merely reproductive organs, but are critical to endocrine, musculoskeletal, behavioural, and anti-neoplastic health.'

The discussion about whether or not to neuter has never been short on myth and misconception. On top of this, we now have all this new and, perhaps somewhat surprising, information to consider. There is always a discrepancy between scientific knowledge and what we actually do and say, simply because it takes a long time for habits to change, and new information to filter down and become common practice. Every dog and cat owner will be faced with the decision either to neuter or leave intact, and certainly deserves to be well informed in that choice.

I am going to tell you what is currently known so that you can make a well-informed decision. This is an area where (surprising) new insights are still emerging, and where everything we (the veterinary profession) thought we knew is being revisited, so some of this information about the potential detrimental

health implications of neutering dogs will be news to many for some years to come. For this reason, I include a list of references on page 217 that you may like to refer to, should you find yourself talking to a fellow dog lover or vet who (understandably) still has some catching up to do.

Research in this area is ongoing, and will undoubtedly have a far-reaching impact on how we approach this topic in the future. If, on the other hand, you feel disinclined to read research into the pros and cons of neutering, and really just want to know what the informed veterinary establishment currently recommends, feel free to skip directly to the relevant information on pages 81 and 87.

Dogs

The routine neutering of dogs is a topic that, to date, has been approached very differently in various parts of the world. In Britain, around two out of three dogs are neutered. In the United States, where stray dogs are a real problem, the American Veterinary Medical Foundation (AVMA) until recently recommended routine neutering of all pet dogs. Indeed, this was practically regarded as a prerequisite of responsible pet ownership. As a consequence, nearly 90% of owned dogs in the US are neutered.

By contrast, consider the situation in Scandinavia. In Norway, routine neutering of dogs (male and female) is outright illegal, and is considered deeply unethical. Only medical conditions qualify for dispensation, meaning that practical considerations (such as two males who fight, or perhaps a male and a female sharing the same household) are not considered legitimate reasons to neuter. In neighbouring Sweden, neutering, while not illegal, is still discouraged on ethical grounds. In Sweden, even though routine neutering is an available option, only around seven percent of all bitches are spayed, and an even smaller

Study findings

From a published study from Oregon State University (2016)
'Canine gonadectomy (neutering) increases the risk of several disorders, including obesity, urinary incontinence, urinary calculi, diabetes mellitus, hypothyroidism, hip dysplasia, cranial cruciate ligament rupture, aggressive and fearful behaviour, cognitive dysfunction syndrome (senility), prostate adenocarcinoma, transitional cell adenocarcinoma, osteosarcoma, hemangiosarcoma, lymphosarcoma and mastocytoma.'

From a published study from the University of California, Davis (2016)
'Being neutered increased the risk for both males and females for hypoadrenocorticism, autoimmune hemolytic anemia, atopic dermatitis, hypothyroidism, inflammatory bowel disease (IBD) and hypothyroidism.'

These quotes are included simply to illustrate that, since the 'Golden Retriever study' of 2013, which focused everyone's attention on the unexpected detrimental health consequences of neutering dogs, a multitude of studies have been and continue to be conducted to shed more light on this issue, and that many more previously unsuspected conditions, such as allergic skin disease, inflammatory bowel disease and hypothyroidism, are now being directly linked to neutering.

percentage of male dogs are castrated, leaving more than 93% (some surveys say 99%) of the Swedish dog population intact.

It is interesting that, while most vets (certainly in Europe) are rightly strongly opposed to the cropping of ears and docking of tails, and other surgical alterations of dogs for cosmetic reasons, many will still neuter a young dog for no particular reason at all.

It is worth pointing out that this discussion is not directly related to the issue of breeding. If your living situation allows for free-roaming dogs who mix with other dogs, you will, of course, have to take this into account. When discussing the pros and cons of neutering for both male and female dogs, I am not discussing population control, but am, instead, focusing entirely on the health risks and benefits for each individual owned and cared-for animal who is NOT intended for breeding. The information in this chapter is aimed at the responsible and well-informed dog owner, who has no intention of letting their dog breed, and who wishes to understand the implications of neutering as it affects the health of their dog. Whether or not to neuter in this privileged situation – that is indeed the question.

Please bear in mind that the advice in this chapter refers to the routine (elective) neutering of healthy individuals. Specific living conditions or health considerations may, of course, decide for or against the neutering of an individual animal.

THE FEMALE DOG

The heat cycle

Most bitches will come into heat twice a year. This is the time of ovulation, so the bloody vaginal discharge from a bitch in heat does not correspond to the menses of human females. The average interval between two seasons is around six months, but intervals of four to eight months are common, and considered completely within normal variation.

The first season is often seen at around six to ten months of age. Small dogs generally mature earlier than large breeds, who may have turned a year old by the time of their first season. An elderly bitch will not go through menopause. Female dogs stay under hormonal influence throughout their lives, although the signs of being in heat may become less clear, and the cycle less regular in old age.

The season lasts around three weeks, during which time the bitch will attract male dogs, who can smell her across long distances. She will bleed during these three weeks, which can be quite a lot, while others bleed less, lick themselves clean, and hardly leave a drop on the floor. Some owners barely notice: some wipe the floor and wash the bedding, and others prefer to make the bitch wear panties for the three weeks to contain bleeding in the house.

The bitch is actually fertile for only a few days, generally during the middle week of the season, but it is impossible to know exactly when she is fertile and when she is safe (assuming you are not intending to breed). For this reason, I absolutely recommend keeping her on a lead at all times when outside of the house for the full three weeks. Even if you have a fenced-in garden or yard and your dog has never before tried to escape, she will suddenly be motivated to do so, just as male dogs from miles away may smell her and choose to break in. It only takes five minutes, so please don't risk it. I have diagnosed plenty of pregnancies with shocked owners who swore that she was not left alone in the garden for a late-night pee for more than five minutes, and absolutely could not have mated. Keep her on a lead, and stay with her whenever she goes outside of the house for those three weeks.

These two issues – cleaning up bloody discharges and having to keep your bitch on a close rein during her seasons – constitute the hassle of having an intact female. These are the practical reasons why spaying may make your life easier. Having said that, we are talking about three weeks twice a year, and most carers come to see it as a natural part of the life of a female dog, rather than a real problem. Of course, things become more complicated if you also have an intact male dog, in which case sending him off to stay elsewhere for a few weeks is often the best solution, if this is possible.

Now, let's look at the health considerations and the options, should you decide that an intact female is not for you.

Spay

Spaying (or sterilisation) is a surgical procedure that permanently removes the female sexual organs. Your dog will become sterile and her seasons will stop. A traditional spay may remove both the uterus and the ovaries (ovario-hysterectomy) or, more commonly today, only the ovaries (ovariectomy). There is no noticeable difference between these two surgical methods, as both remove the ovaries, which stops all hormonal activity.

A newer and less common approach is the ovary-sparing spay, in which the ovaries are left in place, and only the uterus is removed. This procedure still results in infertility, but in all other aspects the bitch will remain hormonally intact.

Regardless of which surgical technique is used, the result of spaying is to render the female permanently infertile. There are injections and implants that will chemically postpone a season, but they are still associated with such a high risk of serious side effects that I can't recommend their use.

Support around surgery

Spaying is always major abdominal surgery. The vet will ask you to withhold food from the evening prior to surgery, and to drop her off at the surgery in the morning. In most cases, you can pick her up again the same afternoon. She will need to rest for a few days, and you will be asked to keep an eye on the wound, and to ensure that she doesn't lick it. The wound should heal completely in under two weeks.

Your vet will provide pain relief to be

continued at home, and may want to check on your bitch during the first week of recovery. For extra support around spaying, see the chapter on surgery, page 199.

Health pros and cons of spaying

See page 82 for more information on the ovary-sparing spay. The following refers to a traditional spay: that is, either an ovario-hysterectomy or an ovariectomy.

The pros ...

By having your bitch spayed, you avoid the hassle associated with seasons, and remove the risk of pyometra (womb infection). There also seems to be a reduced risk of mammary tumours (breast cancer) in neutered compared to intact bitches, although we do not know by how much the risk is reduced, or whether the age of neutering affects this.

These questions have become the focus of renewed and intensive study: for the past 50 years, vets have been quoting figures that came from a single study published in 1969. This study has now been discredited, and the consensus at the time of writing is that we simply don't know as much as we thought we did about the effect of neutering on the risk of breast cancer in dogs. It is a matter of going back to the drawing board. There does seem to be an effect, but we don't know the extent, and we cannot confirm (as previously assumed) that the risk is different in a bitch spayed before the first season as opposed to a bitch spayed much later in life.

... and the cons

The most common side effect of spaying female dogs is development of urinary incontinence, due to the hormonal changes that occur as a consequence of removing the ovaries. Urinary incontinence is rarely seen in intact bitches, but in neutered bitches, as many as one in five develops this problem, which can occur at any time after the surgery,

but most commonly three to five years afterward. It seems that the risk of developing spay incontinence increases when the bitch is spayed when very young (under five months of age).

For the treatment of hormone-dependent urinary incontinence (spay incontinence) in bitches, see page 183.

Other commonly seen side effects are coat changes (purely cosmetic, but a big deal in a show dog), and a tendency to gain weight due to increased appetite and altered metabolism.

As mentioned in the introduction to this section, recent studies have alerted us to a markedly increased risk of several types of cancer and joint disease associated with neutering. That health problems as common and serious as hip dysplasia, elbow dysplasia, and disease of the anterior cruciate ligament of the knee may turn out, in many cases, to be a side effect of neutering is likely to change neutering practices in the future. The possible ill effects are still being investigated as we become increasingly aware that the sexual hormones have a profound effect on the whole body, and are in no way limited to reproduction.

Studies also mention that the immune system seems to be adversely affected by the absence of sexual hormones, possibly causing a higher risk of allergies and immune-mediated disease. One study has even found that neutered animals have a higher risk of adverse effects following vaccination.

Effect of spaying on behaviour

Neutering may reduce aggression toward other bitches. General reactivity, fear and aggression toward people, on the other hand, are more likely to become worse from neutering. Experts specifically point out the importance of avoiding neutering young bitches who have shown any early signs of aggression or dominance toward people, as neutering will most likely exacerbate this behaviour.

Bitch spay: health benefits and risks

Benefits
- *No risk of pyometra (womb infections)*
- *Reduced risk of mammary tumours (breast cancer)*

Risks
- *Risk of urinary incontinence and increased risk of cystitis*
- *Increased risk of joint disease (cruciate ligament disease, hip dysplasia and elbow dysplasia)*
- *Increased risk of several types of cancer (lymphoma hemangiosarcoma, osteosarcoma, mast cell tumour)*
- *Possible increased risk of a range of immune-mediated diseases, such as allergies and auto-immune disease*

It all depends

Making the right decision for each dog is no simple matter. Weighing the benefits against the risks has to include each dog's unique situation, partly because there is so much we now know that we don't know, yet (!), and partly because assessing risk is a complicated business.

Reducing the risk of mammary tumours (as spaying will do) is certainly worthwhile; even more so because mammary tumours are very common in bitches. On the other hand, it is easy to detect mammary tumours. Any owner can learn to feel for them and contact the vet straight away if any lumps or swellings appear in the breast tissue when the bitch is not in season. Breast cancer that is detected early in dogs is rarely fatal, as it can be readily treated.

Compared to breast cancer, the risk of developing other cancer types (significantly increased by spaying), is quite low. However, unlike breast cancer, these cancer types are difficult to detect, and in most cases the diagnosis amounts to a death sentence. To further complicate matters, it appears from recent studies that the effect of spaying varies greatly between breeds. This applies to the cancer risk as well as the effect on joint diseases, such as cruciate ruptures and hip dysplasia. Studies have shown that the effects are dramatic for some breeds, while for others they can't be shown to exist at all. The next few years will undoubtably produce new research to shed light on this area.

What to do?

Firstly, consider *your* situation. Your decision about whether or not to neuter your bitch will depend on factors such as how many dogs you have, and whether you feel up to the task of isolating a bitch in heat. The so-called misalliance injections given to induce abortions after accidental matings carry very high risks, and should not be relied on as an excuse not to keep your bitch from mating. It is a fall-back option only, to be used in real emergencies.

If you can't realistically keep your bitch away from male dogs when she is in heat, it is probably best to have her neutered or, if she is not yet yours, to go for a male puppy instead.

For now, my advice is that if you can handle your bitch being in heat, and feel confident that you can prevent accidental matings, I highly recommend leaving her intact. As long as you regularly check her breast tissue for lumps and swellings, and are aware of the signs of pyometra (page 187), this seems the healthiest option.

If your dog is of a breed (such as Bernese Mountain Dog, Flatcoated Retriever, Golden Retriever, Boxer or Rottweiler) that has an above-average incidence of cancer, at the moment, the consensus among specialists is that leaving her intact is absolutely the safest option. Spaying a Rottweiler will quadruple her risk of bone cancer to a staggering risk of one in four. Your vet should inform you of this: for a veterinary clinic to schedule a routine spay without proper discussion of the risks involved, as was the custom only a few years ago, can have tragic consequences, and is no longer considered an acceptable approach.

On the basis of the knowledge we have today, some bitches simply cannot afford what appears to be a highly increased risk of terminal cancers caused as a direct consequence of spaying.

The ovary-sparing spay

In the ovary-sparing spay (also referred to as OSS, hysterectomy or partial spay), only the womb is removed, and the ovaries are left intact. This is still a fairly unusual option, and one that many vets have never performed, or may possibly not even be aware of.

This procedure is drastically different from the standard surgical spay discussed above. The bitch will become infertile, as she will no longer have a womb, but because the ovaries (sometimes one; sometimes both) remain in place, she will function hormonally exactly like an intact bitch. This means that none of the side effects listed above will apply, as these all result directly from withdrawing the hormonal influence.

After an ovary-sparing spay, therefore, the bitch will have no increased risk of urinary incontinence or coat or temperament changes. In fact, in terms of health – including cancer risks – she will be exactly like an intact bitch in every way, with the one exception that she cannot get pyometra. She still has a full set of hormones, but she can't get pregnant for the same reason that she can't get a womb infection: because she doesn't have a womb.

The surgical incision will be bigger than that required for a normal spay because more precision is needed when removing the uterus (womb) to ensure that no uterine tissue is left behind. In a traditional spay, there is no problem associated with leaving behind a bit of the uterus, as it will not be under the influence of the ovaries, meaning there is no risk of pyometra (womb infection).

As mentioned above, the most modern technique for doing a normal spay even leaves the whole uterus in place, and removes just the ovaries. Without the hormones from the ovaries, the uterus doesn't do a thing; not even become infected.

During the OSS procedure, the surgeon is doing the opposite of what most normal spays do. Instead of removing the ovaries and leaving the uterus (or, as was done historically, removing both), she is removing the uterus and leaving the ovaries. This means that if any uterine tissue is left behind, it will be under the influence of the ovarian hormones, and the dog will run the risk of developing pyometra (this is known as stump pyometra). This cannot happen if the surgery is performed properly, with a big enough incision to visualise the whole of the uterus and make sure that it is tied off very precisely, leaving no tissue behind.

This is the reason why an OSS scar will be much longer than the tiny scar that follows most standard spays performed through keyhole surgery, and why the OSS procedure will be charged at a higher rate than

---

To spay or not to spay?

At the moment, and assuming the owners can manage a bitch in heat and know to look out for signs of breast cancer and womb infection (both treatable conditions), the evidence seems to support keeping your bitch intact or, if choosing to spay, going for a partial spay as the healthier option

a standard spay. Higher precision means a bigger incision, more stitches, and more time.

Assuming that the whole uterus is removed, eliminating the risk of pyometra, mammary cancer is the only increased risk for the bitch with an OSS compared to that of a standard spay (ovarian cancer is so rare that it never justifies removing the ovaries to preclude it). The benefits of an OSS compared to a full spay are the same as the benefits of staying intact (no risk of spay incontinence, no weight gain or coat changes, reduced risk of several cancer types, and reduced risk of hip and knee disease).

Why operate at all?

The only difference in terms of health risks between an intact bitch and a bitch who has had an ovary-sparing spay is that the latter cannot get a womb infection, as she has no womb. I have to say that I struggle with the argument for removing a healthy organ purely to prevent disease. Therefore, the only OSS cases I know as a vet are those where OSS was performed because of a diagnosed womb infection. This is where I see the most relevance for this surgical procedure – in cases where there is a diseased womb but the owners are not interested in neutering because of the associated risks. For these animals, removing the uterus and leaving the ovaries in place is the ideal solution. For anyone else, I would leave the bitch intact and spare her the surgery. It is not as hard as one might think to prevent a bitch from mating, and to look out for signs of mammary tumours and pyometra.

OSS may be the perfect 'middle-ground' for some dogs and their owners, allowing a hormonally-intact bitch who cannot get pregnant. I suspect that this procedure will become popular mainly in areas where keeping animals intact has not been culturally acceptable in the past, and therefore may make some carers uncomfortable. It is

certainly my experience that dog owners and vets who are not used to intact female dogs are overly worried about the dangers of pyometra, whereas vets and dog owners in areas where intact animals are common are simply aware of the risk, and spot the disease if it happens, with the result that deaths almost never occur because of it.

> **Timing may be everything (but in this case it's not yet well understood)**
>
> *Judging by the research available so far, it increasingly appears that the ideal timing of an elective spay is after the bitch has reached sexual maturity – that is, after the first season. Further research that compares statistics from the US (where many are spayed at under eight weeks) to those from most of Europe (where spaying at around six months is the norm) and Sweden and Norway (where spaying is uncommon) will shed more light on this.*

Life after OSS

There are other practical advantages to life with an OSS bitch compared to an intact bitch. Being hormonally completely normal, she will still come into season twice a year, and will still have her false pregnancies, but, because she has no uterus, the bleeding associated with seasons will be negligible, and males will be much less aware of her scent. Apart from this, she will go through a normal season.

Some bitches are very affected during this time; they may become more tired than usual, or attention-seek, and, when the time is right, very keen to get out and find a hot date, just like any other hormonally-intact bitch during her season. Others don't seem to be very affected by their hormones, and, as the discharge is gone, you may hardly notice that she is in heat.

The partially-spayed bitch will be

infertile, but letting her mate is not a good idea. Not only is this a way for diseases to spread and accidents to happen, but there are stories of OSS bitches being mated by much larger dogs, and suffering severe internal injuries.

Timing is everything

If, after careful consideration, you do decide to neuter your female dog, the next important question is how best to time the procedure.

In the US, spaying as early as six to eight weeks, while the puppies are still nursing, is not uncommon; some breeders won't even sell intact female puppies.

Common practice in most other countries is to neuter at five to six months at the earliest, and many choose to wait until the bitch has reached sexual maturity, leaving the spay (or the decision whether or not to spay) until after the first season. This seems a very sensible approach to me, and, based on emerging studies, is looking more and more like the best approach. Science aside, I get a very uncomfortable gut feeling at the thought of neutering babies.

Increasingly, it looks as though we should think twice before neutering at all, but it makes sense to at least allow bitches to mature normally before we intervene with procedures whose implications we are only just beginning to properly understand.

Once a bitch has had her first season (a sign that she has reached sexual maturity), it is important that, should you elect to spay, the procedure is timed to take place between seasons during the period of anoestrus. This means that, if you decide during a season not to let your dog have another, you need to schedule the spay to take place about three months later. She should not be spayed during her season, or during the first two months after the season.

Of course, if your bitch is being neutered for health reasons, perhaps because she has a mammary tumour or a womb infection, you probably can't afford the luxury of carefully timing the surgery; it simply needs to be done as soon as possible.

Spaying during or too close to a season causes hormonal havoc, and can induce an extreme false pregnancy because of the sudden drop in progesterone levels, as described below. In the case of a badly-timed spay, this happens because the ovaries have been removed.

FALSE PREGNANCY

False pregnancy, or pseudopregnancy, is not a disease, but a completely natural phase that affects all intact female dogs to some degree. Some don't show any signs or symptoms of this at all, whilst others are so affected that it becomes a problem for them as well as for their humans.

How does it happen?

Strange as it sounds, a bitch's normal hormonal cycle works in such a way that, after a season, her body cannot tell whether she has become pregnant. Regardless of whether she was mated and got pregnant, was mated but didn't get pregnant, or was never even mated at all, she remains under the influence of the pregnancy hormone progesterone for a long time following ovulation (which happens during the season). If she did become pregnant, there would be a sharp drop in the level of progesterone just before she goes into labour.

This drop in progesterone causes a rise in the hormone prolactin, which stimulates milk production in preparation for the arrival of puppies. If she is not pregnant, the corpus luteum (the area of the ovary that produces progesterone after ovulation) will 'burn itself out.' This typically happens at around 45 to 60 days after ovulation.

What this all means is that there will

be a drop in progesterone around the time of expected birth (when progesterone drops and prolactin rises), whether or not she is pregnant. It is the high level of prolactin experienced when progesterone falls away that causes most of the symptoms of false pregnancy. This could therefore more logically be referred to as false labour.

Why does it happen?

The female dog's hormonal cycle, as described above, is believed to have developed as a result of dogs being pack animals. This clever mechanism ensures that the females in the group will be hormonally synchronised, and will all be feeling motherly (and even be able to produce milk) at the time when puppies are born into the pack. If something happens to a mother, another female can immediately take over. You could say that, whether mated or not, all the females have been 'expecting.'

What are the signs?

The symptoms of false pregnancy vary greatly. Some dogs just seem a little tired, while others are clingy, anxious or restless. Nesting behaviour is very common, which may turn into more or less confused behaviour, such as repeatedly scratching the floor or bedding, and maybe collecting toys or shoes and behaving as though these are puppies. Reluctance to leave the house and abandon the 'puppies' is common.

It is quite usual for a bitch to lose her appetite for a while during this period. The teats generally grow, and there may be milk. This is all completely normal and doesn't require treatment. It will pass after a few weeks.

Why do some bitches suffer from this?

The hormone prolactin is responsible for most of the changes seen during the period of false pregnancy. While all intact female dogs will probably have the same hormonal levels during this period, it seems that some are more sensitive than others to normal hormonal fluctuations, in the same way, I suppose, that some women are much more affected than others by their hormonal cycle.

What can be done about it?

... by you

If your bitch seems depressed or anxious or maybe produces a lot of milk, and you would like to help her get through this phase as easily and quickly as possible, the following steps will help –

• Remove any surrogate 'puppies' (shoes, toys or the like) that she may have adopted
• Activate and distract her. Many dogs will be reluctant to leave the house during this phase but once out will enjoy a walk.
• Increase the amount of exercise for both body and mind in order to keep her distracted, and help her feel tired and relaxed
• Take extra-long and exciting walks, and play lots of games
• Don't worry if she won't eat – in fact, if her appetite is not affected and she is producing a lot of milk, reduce her food by as much as a third, as this will help to dry up the milk. Don't check her milk supply or massage her teats, as this will stimulate milk production

... by your vet

Your vet can prescribe hormones to end this phase immediately, but this is very rarely needed. It will pass on its own. If your dog tends to exhibit strong signs of false pregnancy, this is more than likely (in fact, it is almost guaranteed) to happen again after the next season, and every season after that. It is not normally something they grow out of. If you treat the 'condition' with hormones, this will have to be repeated every time.

Spaying will prevent false pregnancies

permanently, of course, as it removes the ovaries and therefore the normal hormonal cycle, and your dog will no longer have seasons. An ovary-sparing spay will have no effect on false pregnancies, which will continue unabated. Bach flower remedies (page 110) and homeopathy (page 117) are holistic treatment forms that are very helpful if your bitch needs some help through her false pregnancy.

Personally, I think this is a normal part of being a female dog, and do not consider it a reason for neutering. As a homeopath, I know how easy it is to help when someone is unduly stressed by normal hormonal fluctuations. Many vets will recommend neutering as the only permanent solution, simply because they are not familiar with homeopathy.

I urge you to see a vet who specialises in homeopathy before considering such a step.

The risks

It is a common misconception that repeated false pregnancies increase the risk of developing pyometra (womb infection). This is not the case. The only link between the two conditions (inasmuch as false pregnancy can be called a condition) is that they both require intact sexual organs, and they both happen around the same time, during the period following a season.

In fact, there are only two medical conditions you need to be aware of if your

bitch seems out of sorts in the weeks following her season. One is mastitis. This very rarely happens, but, if it should, the symptoms will include a fever, and red, sore, swollen, rock-hard teats (although it is normal for the teats to be swollen, even with milk dripping or running, provided the tissue is soft).

The other condition that could be masked by or mimic a false pregnancy is pyometra. This can happen at any time but is most common during the first two months after a season. Symptoms are lethargy, loss of appetite, increased thirst, and maybe a discharge from the vulva. If you worry that your dog may have pyometra, get her checked out by a vet. It will likely just be false pregnancy that made her lethargic and off her food, but it is better to check when in doubt.

You can read more about the symptoms and treatment of pyometra on page 187.

The bottom line

For female dogs, the current scientific consensus is that the situation is more complex than is the case for male dogs (who are clearly healthier when left intact).

Veterinary opinion is that it is certainly no longer possible to advocate a blanket policy of neutering females, and advice on whether or not to neuter must be given on an individual basis, considering factors such as lifestyle and health risks related to her breed, as well as the carer's ability and willingness to monitor her health and react to signs of pyometra and mammary tumours.

My personal preference is to keep a female dog intact unless there is a strong argument for neutering.

False pregnancy

If your dog is very affected by her false pregnancy, feed her less and distract her with extra games and walks. Don't feel too sorry for her, and don't worry. This is a completely normal phase, and it will pass on its own. If you feel that she needs help, see a vet who specialises in homeopathy: a very effective treatment when it comes to balancing hormones.

THE MALE DOG

A male dog reaches sexual maturity at around five to six months of age. There is no hormonal cycle controlling his sexual urges. If a bitch is on heat, he will generally be keen. Some male dogs seem to have a naturally low sexual drive, and may only sniff curiously if they meet a bitch in heat. Others will whine or howl relentlessly, lose their appetite, and devote their entire focus to escaping in an attempt to join their heart's desire, even if the bitch on heat is several miles away.

A dog's sexual drive is not related to his level of activity or his general temperament.

Castration

Castration is a minor surgical procedure in which the testicles are removed. This makes the male dog permanently infertile, and, because the male hormone testosterone is produced in the testicles, he will no longer have sexual urges, and will not be very affected by bitches on heat, so will be less likely to roam.

Health pros and cons of castration

Almost all intact male dogs will, not unlike the majority of human males, experience some benign prostatic enlargement in middle and old age. This is harmless, and it is treatable if it causes significant discomfort. By contrast, the risk of prostate cancer is negligible in intact dogs. Prostate cancer is a disease of castrated dogs.

Naturally, castrated dogs cannot get testicular cancer, but this is not a major concern in intact dogs, either, as testicular tumours are easy to detect, unlikely to spread, and consequently easy to cure.

As is the case for neutered bitches, new studies show an increased incidence of cancer and joint diseases such as elbow dysplasia, hip dysplasia, and cruciate ligament disease in neutered as compared to intact male dogs.

Effect of castration on behaviour

Castration will only affect behaviour that is directly associated with a male dog's sexual urges, and will not generally calm behaviour as is sometimes assumed. This means that a

Castration: health benefits and risks

Benefits
* A castrated dog will have a reduced risk of benign prostate hyperplasia in old age and, of course, no risk of testicular cancer. There are, however, no overriding health-based arguments for routine castration*

Risks
* Increased risk of joint disease (cruciate ligament disease, hip dysplasia and elbow dysplasia)*
* Increased risk of several types of cancer (lymphoma, hemangiosarcoma, osteosarcoma, mast-cell tumour)*

boisterous, strong-willed young male dog will become easier to control through time and training, not through castration. Yes, if you castrate the above-mentioned unruly young dog, he will be much calmer in six months, but, trust me, this would have happened anyway. It is called maturing and has nothing to do with him becoming a eunuch.

A castrated dog is less likely to insist on stopping every two minutes to sniff and pee when out walking. This is presumably because the comings and goings of the ladies (and the rivals) of the neighbourhood lose importance. He will also be less inclined to stray, assuming that his straying behaviour was (as it often is) inspired by females on heat.

The verdict is in ...

The consensus among veterinary experts is that, on balance, routine castration is not in the interest, health-wise, of the male dog.
Until very recently, vets believed that neutering made our dogs live longer. Evidence now points to the opposite conclusion, and it turns out that, in fact, intact dogs may live longer.

Castration may reduce or eliminate aggressive behaviour that is directly sexually motivated. This means that a castrated male may stop fighting other male dogs, but he will not become any less aggressive toward people, and any aggressive behaviour based on fear, insecurity, over-protectiveness or a general inability to socialise properly with people or dogs will not be improved at all by castration. It may, in fact, have the opposite effect. To repeat – castration will only affect behaviour that is directly sexually motivated.

Behavioural changes

Positive changes in behaviour that may be expected from castration are these: one form of aggression, namely, aggressive behaviour toward other males, may improve, as may any tendency to stray. That's it. Negative changes in behaviour that may occur from castration are increased aggression toward people (including the owners), and increased reactivity (to noise, being left alone, and so on)

Vasectomy

A much less common approach to neutering a dog, vasectomy may have a greater role to play than is usual today. During vasectomy, a small incision is made in the front of the scrotum, and the tube that carries sperm out of the testicles (the vas deferens) is cut. The testicles are left in place, but the sperm can no longer be ejaculated, and so is simply reabsorbed. Because the testicles still function normally, reproductive hormone production isn't affected at all.

A vasectomy leaves the dog intact in all regards concerning both health and behaviour. The only difference is that he will be 'shooting blanks': he will be infertile. Vasectomy may therefore be the solution in areas where it is important to consider population control.

In many European countries, where dogs would never roam free and unaccompanied anyway, this procedure makes little sense, however. If the dog is never going to be allowed to mate (which is certainly the safest approach (one or both dogs could be harmed during unsupervised mating), he may as well be kept intact, and if, for whatever health or behavioural reason, you might want to have him neutered, vasectomy won't do it.

It could be the answer in the US (in areas where free-roaming dogs are common) as a way to keep a dog physiologically intact yet sterile, and it could be a way for shelters and rehoming centres to refrain from neutering. It may also be the answer when keeping a male and a female together without having to neuter either. In this way, they can both be physiologically intact and free to mate without resulting pregnancies. I am not, of course, saying that a vasectomised dog should ever be allowed to roam or mate unsupervised.

Cryptorchidism

A dog is cryptorchid if one or both testicles are retained in the abdomen or in the inguinal canal, instead of having descended into the scrotum during normal development.

The risk of testicular cancer in an undescended testicle is increased thirteenfold compared to that of a normal testicle. Testicular cancer is not normally a great health risk in male dogs, as it is easily detected and slow to spread. In cryptorchid dogs, detection is difficult, and the risk greatly increased. This, together with the fact that cryptorchidism is an hereditary problem (so the dog must not be allowed to breed) has led to a general recommendation that all cryptorchid dogs should be castrated.

If your dog has one retained testicle, and you do not wish to castrate him, there is no reason why you shouldn't be able to simply have the retained testicle removed, and have a vasectomy done on the normal testicle. In this way, your dog will have no increased cancer risk, will be unable to breed (and thereby pass on the trait), and will still be hormonally intact.

Timing

As there is no cyclicity to a male dog's hormones, timing is not really an issue. I suggest leaving your dog intact unless he develops a problem that could be helped through castration. This also ensures that he matures under normal hormonal influence.

This is, at the time of writing, in accordance with current expert advice.

Chemical castration

To achieve a so-called chemical castration, a vet injects a small, hormone-releasing implant under the dog's skin. The implant comes in two sizes, giving a period of testosterone suppression lasting six and twelve months respectively.

In practice, the effect often lasts much longer than the minimum period quoted. The implant inhibits testosterone production, and, once the effect takes hold, the testicles visibly shrink and sperm production ceases. Be aware, though, that viable sperm may remain for up to two months following the injection; some dogs appear to remain fully fertile.

Chemical castration can be a useful way to 'test' the effect of castration on your dog. I find that many dog owners who choose this route express immense relief that the effect is reversible, and are very happy that they didn't immediately go for 'proper' (surgical) castration. It is probably not a good idea to go for repeated implants. If, after the first implant, you wish the effect to be permanent, surgery is a better choice.

CATS

The way in which we keep cats, as with the way in which we keep dogs, differs enormously from one culture to the next. In my native Denmark, everyone seems to agree that the ideal life for a cat is one with freedom to roam. Those who live too close to heavily-trafficked areas or who (for other practical or safety reasons) are unable or unwilling to let their cats roam, will invariably be apologetic, clearly regretting not being able to offer their cat an ideal lifestyle. In complete contrast, letting your cat wander outdoors is considered irresponsible in other parts of the world.

You might imagine that these cultural and geographical differences would affect neutering recommendations, but, actually, they don't. The question of sexuality is quite clear cut when it comes to cats.

Living dangerously

Cats with outdoor access live their lives exposed to two main risk factors: traffic and other cats. Both types of encounter occur predominantly at night, so keeping your cat indoors overnight is a big step toward preventing accidents; another is neutering before the onset of puberty.

Intact male cats stray much further and for longer periods than do neutered male cats or female cats: behaviour that puts them at increased risk of being injured or killed on the road. For both sexes, cat interaction is going to be predominantly sexual or aggressively territorial by nature. Whether they are fighting other cats or having sex, the behaviour carries significant risk of both injury and the transmission of disease. A cat who is neutered before five to six months of age (some are done much earlier; more on that later) will not be mating, and is far less likely to fight.

More than anything else you do for your cats, these two steps – getting them neutered before sexual maturity, and keeping them in at night – will do the most to keep them safe.

Impose a curfew

Cats are, of course, nocturnal by nature, but

adult cats sleep most of the time, and most seem to have no trouble adjusting to a rhythm of going out during the day only. If you use a cat flap, simply set it to 'in only' at some point in the late afternoon, before dinner is served. Once he comes in to eat, there is no going back out that night.

Most cats prefer going to the toilet outside, and can easily hold it until the next morning, but, even if it is rarely used, an indoor litter tray is a good idea.

Safety steps

There are two steps that will go far to ensure a long healthy life for your cat –
- *Don't let a sexually mature cat go outside until they have been neutered*
- *Keep your cat indoors at night*

No sex, please

There is a reason why cats have nine lives. Cats suffer from serious infectious diseases to a much, much greater extent than do dogs, and fighting and mating are the two main ways by which many viral diseases, including feline Aids and leukaemia, are spread.

During the sexual act, the male cat bites the female in the scruff of the neck, which means that she is exposed to semen, blood and saliva, and the risk of disease transmission is therefore extremely high. If you have your cats neutered before they reach sexual maturity, you'll stop the mating completely, and markedly reduce the fighting.

I recommend, when possible, that you keep your kitten confined indoors until the spring after you get him or her. As most kittens are born in the spring and summer, that would make them six to 12 months old. This means that they will be neutered before being introduced to the outside cat population, and has the added benefit of postponing and reducing the need for vaccination. (See the chapter on vaccination on page 42.)

THE FEMALE CAT

In contrast to the female dog, the question of whether or not to neuter is an easy one. Female cats should be neutered, regardless of their living situation.

Her hormonal activity is stimulated by daylight, so sexual activity is centred around the summer months. Depending largely on the time of year, the female cat will come into her first season when she is six to 12 months old. Some cats, particularly pure breeds, can become sexually mature as early as four months of age.

Caterwauling

A queen (female cat) in heat does not go unnoticed, and novice cat owners often contact the vet, believing that there is something seriously wrong with their cat. She will be restless, throwing herself on the floor and rolling around, crying heartbreakingly and incessantly. She will in every way be absorbed by her hormones during this phase, which can be incredibly frustrating to her as well as to anyone in her vicinity.

Cats are unique in that they will ovulate only when mated, and this is what concludes the season. If she is mated and becomes pregnant, kittens will be born two months later, and, while the litter is still nursing, she will come on heat again, ready to start over.

A queen can have three litters in one year. If she is on heat and not mated, she will be back on heat after a few weeks or days, until it almost seems like a constant state; one that quickly becomes unbearable for all concerned, and which won't stop until she is mated or spayed.

If you want her to breed later

If you can't put her out of her misery by having her neutered because you would like her to breed when she gets a bit older, you have a problem without an easy solution. What to do about the almost constant heat until she is old enough to breed or until it suits your planning?

Don't use the contraceptive pill for cats

I'm afraid there's no good answer to the above question. A contraceptive pill is available, but this is – more than any other drug I can think of – just plain bad medicine, whose side effects are potentially deadly: you really don't want to go there. The manufacturer even advises against giving the pill to queens who are intended for later breeding, which completely refutes any justification for its use.

Cats not intended for breeding should be neutered before puberty, and those intended for later breeding will, for the time being, have to endure the intervening misery.

Teaser toms

Breeders sometimes keep a vasectomised male cat who can mate with the females to induce ovulation, and thereby end the heat cycle without a pregnancy. A vasectomised male is, as described for male dogs, hormonally intact but infertile.

For the pet cat, who is just supposed to have a single litter before being neutered, a teaser tom is unlikely to be at hand to solve the problem. This leaves little choice except to endure the seasons, keep her separated from other cats until she is at least one year old, let her have her litter, and then have her spayed when the kittens are about a month old, before her hormonal cycle begins again.

When to neuter

In some parts of the world, kittens are neutered long before they are ready to leave their mother. While I understand the argument that it is crucial to avoid unwanted and therefore homeless kittens, I cannot support the practice of neutering babies. Instead of neutering at less than two months of age, I much prefer leaving them as long as possible, until just before they become sexually mature,

allowing them to turn at least five months old or perhaps more, depending on their lifestyle and the time of year.

To the shelter board that feels it would be irresponsible to rehome intact kittens, I have to say that if you can't trust people to neuter their cat after a few months, how can you hand over an animal to them? This is a basic and obvious requirement for any cat. Once properly informed about the risks of letting mature, intact cats go outside, carers can surely be trusted to take care of their animals?

Unless you are keeping indoor cats for the specific purpose of breeding, there is really no alternative to neutering. As described in this section, it is the only responsible, safe and tolerable choice for your cat, regardless of whether or not she goes outside.

Unlike spayed bitches, spayed female cats don't develop urinary incontinence.

Support around surgery

The vet will ask you to withhold food from the evening prior to surgery, and to drop her off at the surgery in the morning. If she has outdoor access, it is a good idea to keep her inside overnight. Cats have this sixth sense that warns them this is the one morning not to be around.

In most cases, you can pick her up again the same afternoon. She will need to stay indoors and rest for a few days, and you will be asked to keep an eye on the wound and ensure that she doesn't lick it. The wound should heal completely in under two weeks. For extra support around spaying, read the section on surgery on page 199.

THE MALE CAT

It is almost impossible to keep an intact male cat. He would be at greatly increased risk of both accidents and disease, as he would be far more into roaming, fighting, and, of course, mating any un-neutered stray females – sure ways to become infected with one of the many cat viruses. If he is kept indoors, there is a high chance that he will try to escape.

Most intact male cats will, at some point, start urine-spraying to mark their territory. I have, on occasion, met intact male cats living indoors without any problems, but I see it as the exception that proves the rule. Letting a sexually mature tom outside to mix with other cats is deeply irresponsible, both to him, any female cats he impregnates, and the resultant kittens. Keeping him indoors is likely to become an unbearable situation for both of you. Once an intact male cat has matured enough to begin spraying, this behaviour may not stop just because he is subsequently castrated. I recommend castrating him before the unwanted behaviour starts.

Timing of castration

As discussed previously in the section on neutering female cats, I have little sympathy for the practice of neutering kittens while they are still at their mother's teats, and there is certainly no medical argument for neutering six- to eight-week-old kittens. A general anaesthetic at that age, especially when there is no reason for it, puts unnecessary strain on their organs. And why deprive their growing bodies of the chance to mature normally,

especially in light of emerging evidence that sexual hormones play a larger than previously assumed role in normal growth and development? Sexual hormones have a profound influence on the whole body, not merely on reproduction. Yes, we have to de-sex them, but let's leave it as late as we can, letting them mature naturally, until they turn six months old at least, rather than putting them through surgery at six weeks.

There is some discussion about whether early neutering causes narrowing of the urethra in the adult male cat. Studies have indicated that late castration correlates with a bigger urethral diameter. If so, it is certainly another argument for leaving the kittens alone. A blocked urethra is one of the few true emergencies in veterinary medicine: see more about this condition on page 183.

As most kittens are born in the spring or summer, I recommend, when the situation allows, that you keep your young cat inside until the following spring, and have him neutered before you let him out. This way, you have the luxury of leaving him intact for the longest time (just make sure to have him neutered before his first birthday).

If he has outdoor access earlier, have it done before he turns six months old. You do not want him outside after he is sexually mature.

The final stage: old age, natural death or euthanasia

It occurs to me that we experience all the phases of a full life – from birth, growing up and learning how to relate to the world, to illness, joy, comfort, worry, old age and finally death – in a more intense and speeded-up version through our animals. I am tempted to say that, even though it certainly isn't always easy, it is one of the many benefits that come from living with animals. Does sharing our lives with animals perhaps even make us more human?

BIRTH AND DEATH

The beginning and the end of life share many characteristics. Birth and death are both processes that we often experience as dramatic; maybe even traumatic. Under the right circumstances, however, these processes can be both peaceful and positive. Neither can be fully planned or controlled, and how we would ideally like them to happen is a highly personal matter.

Regardless of whether we are talking about giving birth or facing death, and whether animals or humans are involved, I believe that what determines whether we think back on the experience with a feeling of regret or

with peace of mind comes down to this: did we feel powerless and therefore forced to leave the process and responsibility in the hands of 'experts,' or did we feel prepared and informed, able to influence the process and make the choices that felt right for us?

All good things …

We can't change the cruel fact that the natural lifespan of a dog or cat is only one fifth to one tenth that of a human: our pets will age and die before us. It is inevitable. What we *can* affect is how they age and die. I believe it matters greatly how we face this challenge, not only for the sake of our animals, but also for our own sake and for that of our children, who may experience grief for the first time when they lose a beloved dog or cat. How we approach this last phase of our animal companion's life very much determines how we think back on them in years to come. It also reflects our fears and feelings about our own mortality. You may even choose to see it as an invitation to examine your approach to this matter, which is difficult for most of us.

I have known pet owners who felt this last phase to be so traumatic that they vowed never to have another animal, but I also know families who cherish the memory of their friend in his last days of life, looking back on a beautiful and dignified end to a good life.

Euthanasia

In most countries, ending a human life on compassionate grounds is a crime. The general view on putting animals to sleep when they are ill or old is very different. I do know vets who find the procedure irreconcilable with their personal ethics, and who refuse to euthanise an animal, regardless of the situation. In my experience, however, most vets come to look very lightly on the ending of a life.

The option to euthanise is a welcome safeguard against pain and suffering when there is no hope of recovery, but this power over life and death comes with a responsibility for which most of us are not prepared. It is not uncommon to leave the decision to the vet. Is it the right thing to do? Many, including many veterinarians, would say that, in this situation, the vet is the expert: the one who holds the answers and is best suited to make the decision.

I don't agree.

A question of choice

I feel that euthanasia for people should be a more readily available option, and that a natural death for animals could be far more common, but this is not about my feelings. It is about each of us being able to make a personal choice that enriches an important phase of our lives

Natural death

If your grandmother is nearing the end of life, you expect her to die a natural death. She may be in hospital, she may be on medication, but, in most cases, the question of euthanasia is never even considered. If your old dog is nearing the end of her life, however, in many parts of the world this will almost invariably happen by means of a deadly syringe. Why the difference?

Is it okay to be old?

Your dog is growing old. He sleeps most of the time. He can only manage short, slow, tottering walks. He has to content himself with watching when the next generation plays, and he is in every way a far cry from the ball-playing, super-active and athletic individual he was when he was younger.

But isn't that how it's supposed to be? Couldn't the same be said for your granddad?

We may find it difficult to witness the decline that is a natural part of growing old (especially when it happens over the space of only a few years), but is it defensible to deprive someone of their last years because we feel that they should always be in their prime, and are saddened, and maybe challenged, by this constant reminder of mortality? No one is supposed to be in their prime forever. No dog is four years old forever. Even so, the perception that euthanasia is the kindest option as soon as decline sets in is not uncommon.

Euthanasia as an option to prevent suffering is certainly a blessing, but I believe that we must be careful not to lose sight of the gravity of the act of killing. We should not find ourselves in a moral landscape where we cannot tolerate an ill, old or even dying animal without automatically reaching for the syringe.

Vets are humans, too

Euthanasia can be a way to maintain an illusion of control: the vet may feel that she still had the situation under control; was able to stay in charge and offer a solution. We are all powerless in the face of death, but we prefer not to dwell on that fact, so stepping back and allowing a natural process to take place can be difficult.

Decisions about life and death go to the core of who we are and are not simply a matter of medical expertise. Loss and death are inevitable parts of life. To me, in the end it matters not so much whether an animal is euthanised or dies a natural death – either can be right in a given situation – what matters, I think, is that it is *your* process. Both your dying animal and you should be fully supported so that, whatever happens, it feels right to you now and when you look back on it in years to come. Of course, it is a sad, sad time, but it can also be an important and meaningful time if we relinquish the pressure, panic, guilt, denial, regret and expectation of control, and are able to say goodbye and let go.

When the experts don't have all the answers

Your vet is, as always, your all-important ally during the last phase of your animal's life. He or she can diagnose and treat symptoms of illness, advise you on appropriate nursing care for your old or dying animal as their needs change, and help assess whether your animal is in pain and provide pain relief if needed. They can prepare you for what to expect. What they can't do, in most cases, is tell you the right thing to do when it comes to the hardest decision, that of life and death.

The last days

Of course, animals must never be allowed to suffer needlessly. In some cases, it is obvious that the quality of life is unacceptable, and not likely to improve, in which case the decision to euthanise is clearly the right one. Sometimes it happens that a dog or a cat simply doesn't wake up one morning, and there is no decision to be made.

In most cases, however, there will be a period of heart-wrenching deliberation when an animal nears the end of life. You take it one day at a time, watching the decline, hoping in equal measure not to have to make the decision to end it, and not to have to live afterward with the regret of having left it too long.

Talk things through with your veterinarian, with your friends, family, and anyone else who knows you and your dog or cat. At the end of the day, accept that the decision is yours. It is a heavy one. It may seem tragic, but it helps to remember that what is happening is exactly what it supposed to happen. It may be helpful to try and imagine looking back on this period a year from now, visualising how your choices will seem to you then, when distanced from the acute grief and fear that may cloud your vision now.

There is no question that we will lose our animal companions. Our power, at the most, extends only to the how and when.

Nobody dies of old age

As described above, euthanasia can be one way for both carer and vet to maintain the illusion of control in the face of terminal illness. Denial is another. The problem, as I see it, is that nobody dies of old age. Old age is simply not a diagnosis. What happens, when the end approaches, is that we (and our animals) experience organ failure or become terminally ill. The cause of death for a 12-year-old dog or a 16-year-old cat will by definition never be old age, but may be cancer, pneumonia, or kidney or liver failure. Putting very old animals through major surgery or chemotherapy, feeling that they have tragically fallen ill and that we have to save them, is another common reaction to pending death. Tests and treatments will be available, even when it is absolutely clear (from the disease process or simply the age of the animal) that a cure is impossible and death is the certain outcome.

I frequently meet people who are desperate and determined to beat death, whatever they must put their animal through to attempt it. Very often, a simple dialogue about what is actually supposed to happen at this stage can ease their fear and panic,

Euthanasia: consider this

- *Old age is a natural part of life; not an unpleasant phase to be skipped*

- *Everybody will have a point of view, and this includes those with no insight into your situation!*

- *You are allowed to change your mind at any time. Keep an open mind. No one can plan death*

- *It makes no sense to wish for a natural death while going ahead with steroid treatment or force-feeding. Tell your animal it's okay to die*

- *Take one day at a time*

- *Sleep on it. In most situations, you can take a day to consider. The right decision is rarely taken under pressure*

- *Putting your thoughts on paper is a great way to see things more clearly. Write a list of pros and cons. What is the worst that could happen if you followed plan A or plan B? Which would you not be able to live with?*

- *If you choose euthanasia now or later, it can happen peacefully and calmly in your own home. Ask about this beforehand, so that your vet will be prepared when you make the call*

and dramatically change the way that carers perceive the situation, as well as the treatment choices they make. We are not supposed to beat death.

The only aspects we can sometimes affect, when a very old animal becomes terminally ill, is whether death occurs a few months sooner or later, and whether the last part of life is lived in relative comfort, or coping with drug side effects or recovering from surgery. I don't believe that animals share our fear of death, yet, illogical as it may be, fighting to avoid death at any cost is very often our instinctive reaction. As we learn to deal with the reality that it can't be done (as our animals, even as they leave us, often help us to do), making the right decisions in each case becomes much easier.

To me, birth and death are both special and important times that I, as a vet, am privileged to be invited to share. I have often noticed that the presents, flowers and letters of gratitude that all vets receive come not from the owners of very ill animals who were cured, but from owners who were supported through, and in the end felt enriched by, the important process of saying goodbye to their beloved companion.

PART TWO
From herbs to homeopathy

As a young vet student anticipating the job of my dreams, my expectations were very clear: my role in the veterinary clinic would be finding out what was wrong with my patients. Once a diagnosis had been reached, the correct treatment would cure the patient.

Today, I see how naive that was. I actually think most vets and doctors are confronted during their first years in practice with the difficult realisation that most of their time is spent managing disease rather than curing it. Whether we are talking about sick animals or sick people, the majority of patients are never cured. The limitations of your chosen profession can be a hard pill to swallow after years of committed study.

The second part of this book looks at the limitations of conventional veterinary medicine, and explores the principles underlying holistic (so-called alternative) treatment methods.

The conventional approach treats the illness; the holistic approach treats the patient.

What does it mean to be holistic?

Who can legally treat animals?

In the UK, as in most of Europe, only qualified vets are allowed to diagnose and treat animals, and this applies to conventional and alternative treatments alike. In a few cases (notably osteopathy and physiotherapy), a practitioner who is not a vet is allowed to treat an animal, provided the animal is first examined by a vet who diagnoses the problem and recommends osteopathy or physiotherapy as a suitable treatment. It may seem bizarre that animals are better protected than humans in this regard, as alternative practitioners who treat humans are generally not required to hold medical degrees. Nevertheless, animals, being less able to communicate their symptoms or give their consent, benefit greatly from this added protection.

The potential downside to this restrictive regulation could be a lack of qualified practitioners. Luckily, a large number of vets hold further qualifications in holistic treatment modalities such as homeopathy and acupuncture. At the end of the book, you will find the information you need to locate them.

In some parts of the world, practitioners with qualifications in alternative therapies but without veterinary degrees are allowed to treat animals. Find out what the rules are in your country and contact the appropriate governing bodies to ensure that your practitioner is properly trained, licensed and insured. If your animal is ill and you want him to be treated by someone who is an authority in their field but not a vet, first consult your vet to ensure a correct diagnosis. A medical diagnosis is always the first step, regardless of which treatment is to follow.

Alternative to what?

Conventional medicine, as it is taught in medical schools to both vets and doctors, takes a very mechanistic view of the patient. The immensely complex living body is broken down into parts, much like a car or a dishwasher. You learn how the different parts work, and when there is a problem you try to locate the bit that is broken, and fix it. Is it the pump or the wiring: the heart or the nervous system?

Many vets and doctors later specialise in specific organ systems. You may have noticed how our hospitals, and increasingly our veterinary referral centres, are organised into departments looking separately at our various parts: gastro-intestinal disease, heart and lung disease, and so on. If a patient doesn't fit into any of the boxes, as is often the case, he can find himself passed from one department to the next without ever meeting anyone able to look outside the box at the bigger picture or the whole patient.

Why does chronic disease exist?

In some situations, the conventional approach described above is an adequate and appropriate way to treat disease. This is especially true in cases of accidents and emergencies, such as severe acute disease or surgical procedures. In many cases, however, this approach simply does not lead to a cure.

　　The large number of people and animals who have to live with a chronic condition are clear examples of this. The term *chronic* means that the illness is long term, and often the patient lives with the same condition for years, and isn't expected to be cured. Ever. This is because the tools available through conventional medicine – the conventional toolbox – don't hold the answer for these patients.

received has clearly not been able to deal with the root of the problem.

The right tool for the job

If the only tool you have is a hammer, every problem looks like a nail. We might turn that expression around and ask: if you have been hammering away for months or years and the effect is temporary at best, is it perhaps time to try a different tool?

　　The more tools the vet or doctor has at her disposal, the better the chance she will be able to cure the patient. It is never a matter of preferring conventional medicine or alternative medicine, but rather of using the approach that works best in any situation. Let me be clear that it is in no way my intention to disregard or undermine conventional medicine or, indeed, vets who practice only conventional medicine. I merely wish to point out that, in those situations, for those conditions and for those patients for whom conventional medicine has

Complementary co-operation

It is never a question of choosing between conventional and alternative healthcare. Use the best of both worlds. Different methods of treatment have different strengths and weaknesses. Remember that, regardless of how your animal is to be treated, the first step always consists of a thorough examination to determine what is wrong. A diagnosis is always the first step

Often, carers will be told by their vet that the disease is incurable, and can only be 'managed' with symptomatic treatment. We could be talking here about the dog with recurring allergic skin problems who needs repeated courses of steroids or antibiotics to keep flare-ups at bay, or the cat who suffers from repeated episodes of cystitis. These are the patients who may benefit from an entirely different approach, as the treatment they have

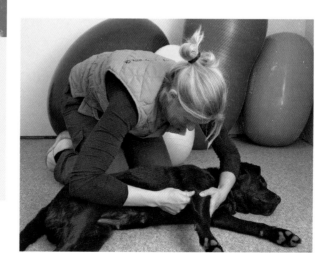

Complete and whole

Holism: the idea that an individual should be viewed as a whole, and not as a collection of parts

not provided an answer, there are alternatives that deserve to be much more widely used.

What alternative?

What exactly are these alternatives that I keep referring to? What *is* alternative medicine?

You may immediately make certain associations when you hear the term. Does alternative simply cover everything that the conventional GP or local vet doesn't provide? Is it feel-good medicine? Something that you like to believe in, or maybe something you choose *not* to believe in? Something less efficient; perhaps only suitable for minor ailments?

The definitions and perceptions are many and varied. The point I wish to make is that the term itself is nonsensical and tainted by association. Alternative? Alternative to what?

The holistic view

Let's define what we're talking about in a way that describes what alternative medicine is rather than what it isn't, or as relative to something else. To this end, let me introduce a different term: instead of 'alternative' medicine, let's talk about 'holistic' medicine. I am not simply mincing words. There is an important point to be made here.

The opposite of holism may be defined as reductionism: a term that describes a treatment approach based on the notion that any individual can be viewed simply as a collection of parts, and that, for example, one case of epilepsy or cystitis will not be fundamentally different to another case of epilepsy or cystitis. This is, in other words, the conventional approach to medicine.

Now that we have defined the two approaches to medicine – holistic (or so-called alternative) and reductionistic (or conventional) – let us examine the differences. They are far-reaching.

Treat the patient, not the disease

A conventional vet or doctor will base her treatment entirely on the diagnosis. It is a simple flowchart. Once you know what the illness is, the treatment for this follows. Individual traits, such as the personality of the patient, are completely irrelevant.

I don't mean to imply that conventional practitioners are not interested in their patients, or don't care about their wellbeing: I simply mean that the treatment is based on the diagnosis alone, and nothing else is relevant in that context. Ten very different individuals with the same diagnosis will receive the same treatment.

In complete contrast, a holistic vet or doctor will base her treatment on the individual

Holistic (alternative)	Reductionistic (conventional)
Focus on the individual	Focus on the diagnosis
Symptoms are important information	Symptoms constitute the problem
Leads to a higher level of health	Eliminate symptoms
Stimulates the inherent self-healing ability	External influence to eliminate symptoms

traits of the patient, and the diagnosis is only one of many factors taken into account when choosing the appropriate treatment for each one. Differences in personality, nuances in symptoms, and a number of other factors will often mean that ten patients suffering from the same condition will be cured by ten different treatments. The treatment must suit the patient and reflect their unique reaction to their disease. This is why most holistic vets will spend an hour or more taking the case of a new patient, while most conventional vets can gather all the information they need in the standard 15-minute consultation.

It takes time to gather the information that is so crucial to a holistic, individualised approach. It is necessary to know the patient in order to pinpoint the exact treatment that will address the imbalance at the root of illness in each case. When compared to simply wanting to supress a bothersome symptom, this is a comprehensive and ambitious approach.

Let me emphasise that, when I discuss the limitations of the conventional, reductionistic approach, I am criticising that whole approach to medicine, not the individual veterinary surgeon. The vet who prescribes steroids or other immuno-suppressive drugs to an allergic dog or cat is, of course, completely aware that she is doing nothing more than suppressing symptoms for a while until the side effects set in. Conventional vets are fully aware that symptomatic treatment will never be able to cure the problem, and they are very often deeply frustrated by not being able to do more.

Different approaches

The conventional vet sees the symptom as the problem and treats to eliminate it.
The holistic vet sees the symptom merely as an indication of a deeper imbalance that must be addressed

What is a symptom – the problem or the road to cure?

As we have just discussed, the emphasis on an individual approach constitutes a main difference between holistic and conventional treatment. Another important difference is the way in which the practitioner perceives symptoms. While we tend to see symptoms as problems, they are, in fact (at least initially), an appropriate response to a problem or threat. We may go to the doctor to take away the itch, the pain or the diarrhoea. However, these symptoms are signs that the body is trying to address a problem. When we cut or burn ourselves, we feel pain so that we will move away from a source of danger. We develop diarrhoea, fever, sneezing and coughing in an attempt to expel invading bacteria that threaten our health. The body generally knows what it is doing. We should listen and help rather than fight against it.

The conventional vet tends to equate the symptoms with the problem, and will treat merely to supress those symptoms. This approach leads to what we call symptomatic relief. The holistic vet, on the other hand, will ask very detailed questions about the patient's symptoms, seeing them as, in a sense, the body's way of talking to us. She will use all the insight and information that she has gathered (partly by analysing the symptoms) to understand the underlying imbalance and, through a very gentle and highly specific treatment, help the organism to heal itself.

Let me illustrate all of this with a favourite story.

Instead of a person or a dog, imagine that our patient is a car, busily driving along the motorway. This car is zooming along, enjoying life, when one day it suddenly develops a symptom – a frustrating and distracting symptom. Let's say that the oil light starts flashing, distracting the driver and decreasing the general quality of life for the car.

If this were you or me or, indeed, my cat, the symptom might be itchy eczema or diarrhoea, but, for the car in our story, it is a flashing light. Symptomatic relief in our situation might be a steroid cream for the eczema or anti-peristaltic drugs to stop the diarrhoea. The equivalent treatment for the car would be covering the oil light with black tape. It is quick, it is easy, it works immediately and it stops the symptom from bothering us. It does not, however, take the symptom seriously or in any way address the reasons why the symptom may have occurred in the first place.

For a while, this symptomatic relief will work very well. The diarrhoea may return and need another course of treatment, the eczema likewise, and the tape may come off, needing a new piece in its place, but, all-in-all, the treatment will be effective – at least for a while.

Inevitably, at some point down the road, the car will develop other and more serious symptoms from a different part of the 'body.' There may be smoke, coughing, and a complete inability to go on when the engine begins to suffer from the poor choice of ignoring the signals at an earlier stage.

The holistic practitioner sees this story repeated all the time when, for instance, eczema is repeatedly suppressed in a dog or cat who then goes on to develop epilepsy or asthma.

How could we have provided holistic care for the car? Well, instead of simply suppressing the offending symptom, a little more time and energy could have been expended. The car would need to pull over, and the root of the problem identified. Once the imbalance had been appropriately addressed, the oil light would have stopped flashing – without needing any direct attention at all. The symptom was not the problem and didn't need to be stopped. It was merely an indication that help was needed.

It is worth noting that, as the car continues its journey, it is in better shape for the road ahead than it was before the lamp ever began flashing. This is a common observation from patients receiving holistic treatment. Often other complaints, which weren't even mentioned during the initial consultation, clear up as well. Carers often comment that their dog or cat seems years younger, and has started playing again in a way that they haven't seen since long before the onset of the illness they sought treatment for.

Holistic treatment affects the whole individual at a deep level, and the effect is often astounding. 'We forgot that he used to bring toys to us' and 'We just assumed that she was getting older' are typical comments from carers after animals have received holistic treatment. They are nice confirmations that, rather than merely suppressing an offending symptom such as an itch or a recurring cough, the treatment has had a deep-acting healing effect.

All or nothing

Individuality and totality are the two cornerstones of holistic treatment. The diagnosis is taken into account but never forms the sole basis for treatment. The practitioner is interested in information about all aspects of the patient, not just the offending symptoms. The treatment must match each individual patient to fit their specific picture: only then is it possible to cure the otherwise incurable

HOLISTIC TREATMENT METHODS

While the major holistic treatment forms share the common principles of individuality (treating the patient, not the disease) and totality (looking at the whole picture, not just the complaint), there are, of course, differences in their application and suitability to different species, and for different conditions.

The following describes the major holistic modalities and their use in dogs and cats. All of these were initially developed for the treatment of people, and have since been adapted for the benefit of animals.

HERBAL MEDICINE

Two different herbal traditions
There are two main traditions of herbal medicine: Chinese herbal medicine and Western herbal medicine. Both were developed primarily for the treatment of humans many centuries ago, and they are equally beneficial in the treatment of animals.

When to see a herbalist
Chinese herbs are often used alongside acupuncture treatments as part of TCM (traditional Chinese medicine). In the hands of a vet trained in TCM, this approach can be used to treat most illnesses. The acupuncture points and the herbs used will be chosen according to a classical five-element analysis, according to the principles of TCM, to suit the individual patient.

Western herbs are often used in a way that is more directly based on the disease to be treated or the organ affected. I tend to regard Western herbal medicine as a link between conventional medicine and the other, more energy-based holistic treatment forms described in this section.

This is hardly surprising, as Western herbal medicine formed the basis of conventional medicine as we know it today. A herbalist (sometimes also referred to as a phytotherapist) would point out that, while her approach in many ways resembles that of the conventional doctor (using medicine in material doses, and selecting the treatment based on the organ to be supported or the disease process to be stopped), using the whole plant or plant part as it appears in nature, rather than a chemically synthesised version of the active ingredient, is a different practice altogether.

While the historical link between Western herbal medicine and conventional medicine makes herbs easily applicable by most practitioners ('This is good for the liver,' is an approach that immediately fits the mindset of most vets), many herbalists will still take a much more holistic approach, looking for patterns in each case before choosing the corresponding herbal treatment.

An increasing number of veterinary products contain Western herbs, aimed at supporting dogs and cats with chronic disease such as digestive problems or chronic liver, bladder or kidney disease. These supplements (nutraceuticals) are easy to use and often make a profound difference to a chronically ill animal. See page 211 as well as the chapters on specific illnesses for some of my favourite herbal supplements.

Herbal medicine around the world
Chinese herbs are used widely by holistic vets, who will often use herbal mixtures in conjunction with acupuncture in dogs and cats. While acupuncture treatments at regular intervals will provide immediate relief, herbs administered at home, between sessions, support and maintain the effect, and can reduce the frequency of acupuncture treatments.

Western herbs are increasingly used in veterinary medicine, based on either an individual consultation with a veterinary herbalist who selects the appropriate treatment for each animal, or, perhaps more commonly, as organ support selected in a more conventional approach that depends on the problem to be treated rather than individual analysis of the patient. A vast range of products is available. See details on page 211 and in the chapters on specific illnesses.

Herbal or homeopathic?

Herbal medicine is easily confused with Bach's flower essences or with homeopathic medicine, not least because many of the same plants are used, but it is important to appreciate the differences. Homeopathy and Bach flower remedies are both energetic treatments, meaning that it is not possible to poison or in any way harm a dog or cat by giving a homeopathic remedy or a Bach flower remedy. This is not the case with herbal medicine. Although 'natural' and beneficial when used correctly, herbal medicine involves giving substances that can be toxic in the wrong doses, or if given to the wrong patient. Always seek professional advice before giving herbs to your dog or cat.

The treatment

Herbal treatments will vary depending on whether Chinese or Western herbs are given, and on the condition of the animal. In most cases, your veterinary herbalist will not recommend the use of a single herb, but will instead prescribe a mixture of carefully chosen herbs that complement one another and suit the patient.

Ask your vet for advice or for a referral, and see page 215 for help in finding a veterinary herbalist.

Duration of treatment

The length of treatment will naturally depend on the condition to be treated. As a general rule, do not give your animal herbs on a long-term basis without good reason for doing so. If your dog or cat has a chronic and incurable condition, such as permanent liver or kidney damage, your vet may prescribe lifelong herbal treatment as part of their care. I do not recommend administering herbs long term as a general booster to a healthy individual or in the absence of a diagnosis, as this could inadvertently do harm.

The medicine

Chinese herbs are generally supplied by your herbalist as ready-made mixtures of dried herbs. They can be mixed with a tasty treat to mask any bitter taste.

You can, of course, grow your own herbs, and either use the fresh herb or make tea from fresh or dried herbs. This is great fun, but it is rarely how herbs are used for medicinal purposes. Apart from issues of practicality, it is impossible to be sure of the concentration of the active ingredient, and therefore of the correct dosage. Most herbalists buy their medicines from suppliers who must document a standardised content of their product. Most medicinal herbs are either dried or extracted in alcohol in the form of a tincture. Dried herbs may be made into tea or given as powder, capsules or tablets.

Buying your herbal product from a reputable firm is the only way to ensure that the herbs were grown and harvested in a sustainable manner, that the botanical classification is correct, and that the concentration of active ingredients has been verified. If you use a veterinary product, testing will have been done to ensure that the product is safe for dogs and cats, and a dosage guide will be included.

EXAMPLES OF COMMONLY USED WESTERN HERBS

Calendula (marigold)

Calendula tincture is so useful that it belongs in every household. Use it topically (on the skin) as an antiseptic. Calendula is also available for topical use in many creams and oils. While these are great for humans, they are, generally speaking, not a good idea for dogs and cats as creams stick to the hair and can encourage licking.

Calendula tincture diluted in water,

however, is a perfect wash or compress that will soothe any rash and help to heal any wound or abscess. It has unrivalled healing and antiseptic properties, and belongs in every home for the treatment of minor wounds, cuts and rashes in humans and animals alike.

See more on the use of calendula tincture to treat wounds on page 151.

Crataegus (hawthorn)

Crataegus has a beneficial effect on the heart, and is often given as a tincture to dogs or cats with heart disease.

This may affect the need for conventional medication, however, and should always be administered with veterinary supervision.

Echinacea

Echinacea is famed for its immune-boosting properties. I rarely use it long term, preferring instead other, more potent approaches to help patients with serious immune-related disease. Echinacea is invaluable, however, when used in the short term to treat or prevent acute infection.

For the sneezing cat or the dog with kennel cough, daily doses of echinacea will support other treatments, and help limit the disease.

Slippery elm

Slippery elm, much like psyllium husks, forms a protective gelatinous layer that protects the intestinal wall. It is of great value in the short or long term until a more lasting cure is found for anyone with digestive sensitivity and a tendency to diarrhoea.

See the section on supplements on page 211.

Euphrasia (eyebright)

Euphrasia is a traditional remedy to soothe irritation of the surface of the eye (the cornea). Dogs and cats who have a tendency to develop conjunctivitis, and may need their eyes cleaned daily, can benefit from euphrasia eyedrops. This can make a big difference, for instance, to dogs of the Spaniel type who have excessively droopy skin around the eyes, and to many short-nosed breeds who may have blocked or underdeveloped tear ducts, leading to constantly gunky eyes or reddish tear stains under the eyes.

Garlic

Many claims are made regarding the almost magical properties of garlic, and this is an example of the need to be very careful when extrapolating from humans to animals.

All plants belonging to the onion family (including garlic, spring onion and onion) are, to some degree, toxic to dogs and cats. The level of sensitivity varies, but while some dogs seemingly tolerate daily garlic supplementation, others have died from the toxic effect of garlic to their red blood cells.

Why risk it? No dog or cat needs daily administration of garlic to stay healthy. I do not support the popular trend of giving garlic to repel parasites; in fact, my advice is to avoid products containing garlic. If your animal has benefited from homeopathic treatment, the effect can easily be antidoted by garlic, so always carefully study the label of any food or supplement to make sure that it does not contain garlic.

Silymarin (milk thistle)

Silymarin, an extract from the seeds of milk thistle, has strong liver-protecting properties. I recommend the use of silymarin for anyone who has been diagnosed with liver disease, as well as in cases of poisoning, or when there is suspicion or risk of poisoning.

This may be the case in animals who require ongoing treatment with drugs that carry a high risk of side effects affecting the liver. Epileptic animals receiving phenobarbitone are the classic example. For these patients, if their seizures cannot be stopped without phenobarbitone, giving milk thistle alongside this anti-epileptic drug can protect the liver from side effects.

Most vets now stock one of several available commercial supplements (nutraceuticals) containing silymarin, often together with other liver-protecting compounds. The benefit of such products to animals suffering from liver disease is well documented.

'It's natural, so it must be good'
There seems to be an exploding market in pet supplements. Herbal products, especially, are available in all forms and combinations. Many of these, it seems, are not aimed at treating specific problems, but promise to be 'beneficial' in a very vague sense. While many are harmless, some are not. The fact remains that herbs should not be given to any animal without the advice of an holistic vet.

Side effects
It is easy to assume that if a product is 'natural' it must be safe. Some compounds are metabolised very differently in animals than in humans, and, when it comes to the use of herbs in animals, this means that we can never simply extrapolate about safety – or indeed dosage – from experience based on human treatment. If a product has not yet been tested on animals, we simply lack insight into its effect, dosage and toxicity. Cats, particularly, are notoriously sensitive, and may react badly to substances that are safe in humans and dogs.

The origin of herbal medicine
Plants have been the basis for medicine for most of human history. Today's modern medicine has developed directly from Western herbal medicine, as pharmaceutical drugs are largely derived from the medicinal plants of the past. It is impossible to know when animals first received herbal treatment, thought it was undoubtedly several thousand years ago.

Mode of action
Western herbal medicine is the foundation of conventional medicine as we know it. Many of the herbal remedies that have been used for centuries, if not millennia, are still used to treat the same conditions, albeit now in a form that is chemically synthesised by the pharmaceutical industry.

There is no common principle or mode of action underlying Western herbal medicine. As in modern medicine, where the active ingredient is given in an isolated form and often chemically synthesised, the pharmacological mode of action varies from one ingredient to the next, and for some medicines it remains poorly understood.

HERBAL MEDICINE SUMMARY
- There are two main schools of herbal medicine: Western herbs and Chinese herbs
- Herbs can be toxic or have side effects in some patients. Use under professional guidance
- Strong-tasting herbs, such as garlic, may antidote homeopathic treatment

ACUPUNCTURE

When to see an acupuncturist
A vet who has been trained in traditional Chinese medicine (TCM) will be able to apply acupuncture in the treatment of almost any condition, often combining needling with the use of Chinese herbs.

Perhaps more commonly, acupuncture is used as the holistic treatment of choice for pain relief in musculoskeletal conditions. It is indicated in practically all cases of osteoarthrosis, whether due to elbow dysplasia, hip dysplasia or spondylosis (osteoarthrosis of the back), or perhaps secondary to an old knee injury. In these very common conditions, acupuncture can significantly reduce the need for conventional pain relief.

Acupuncture can also stimulate nerve tissue, aiding recovery after an accident or a prolapsed disc. Other conditions, ranging from epilepsy to non-healing wounds, are also commonly treated by veterinary acupuncturists.

Acupuncture has played a significant role in the management of skeletal pain in ageing dogs for many years. It is less commonly used to treat cats, but, as veterinary surgeons are becoming increasingly aware that cats suffer skeletal pain to a much greater extent than previously assumed, it is certainly worth considering acupuncture for any cat displaying chronic lameness or stiffness, either following an accident or simply due to ageing. It is amazing how many cats are happy to accept having needles inserted.

Acupuncture around the world

Acupuncture is probably the most established form of holistic treatment. Vets all over the world use acupuncture in the treatment of small animals as well as horses and farm animals. Some are trained in the full TCM approach to disease diagnosis and treatment, often incorporating Chinese herbs. Others take a more Western or pathological approach, focusing primarily on pain relief in musculoskeletal disorders.

From a legal point of view, acupuncture is viewed as a surgical procedure in most countries, meaning that only qualified veterinary surgeons are allowed to carry out this treatment. See page 215 for advice on finding a veterinary acupuncturist.

The acupuncture session

The vet inserts very fine needles into carefully chosen acupuncture points located along meridians all over the body. The insertion is not painful, and the treatment is generally tolerated well by most dogs and cats. Typically, the needles will be left in position for 10 to 30 minutes, during which time the patient often visibly relaxes as the effect is felt.

Other techniques involve stimulating each point more vigorously with a needle for a few seconds, and then removing the needle before moving on to the next point. Less commonly, the vet may use electric stimulation or other means of stimulating the acupuncture points.

Duration of treatment

Depending, naturally, on the nature of the problem being treated, most chronic conditions will require ongoing acupuncture treatment. Many acupuncturists start with an initial series of weekly treatments for the first month or so, before assessing the individual's response to acupuncture. At this stage, it is often possible to increase the time between treatments, maybe settling on a top-up session every couple of months.

Many animals with chronic arthritic conditions will require lifelong treatment to maintain the achieved effect.

'Permanent acupuncture' with gold-bead implants

Gold-bead implants can be a cost-effective alternative to repeated acupuncture treatment for an animal suffering from a chronic condition.

I generally suggest treating animals with acupuncture first to establish that they respond well to this form of treatment. If, after a few months of acupuncture treatments, the effect is good but the treatment needs to be repeated more often than is practical for the carer, gold-bead implants can be the ideal solution.

Instead of repeated stimulation for 20 minutes with an acupuncture needle at weekly or monthly intervals, as in traditional

If at first ...

Walther was an eight-year-old Labrador suffering from hip dysplasia. His carer, an elderly woman who also suffered from severe arthritis, had herself experienced immense pain relief from gold-bead implantation, and from this unique perspective she wanted the same relief for her dog. Walther had the procedure done at a local veterinary hospital but, sadly, showed no sign of improvement. A year later, fully determined that Walther must be able to benefit to the same life-changing degree that she had experienced, Walther's carer took him to another veterinary surgeon with many years' experience in traditional acupuncture, as well as in gold-bead implantation. It was second time lucky for Walther, who responded quickly and profoundly to this subsequent treatment. As the referring vet, I found that this nicely illustrated that, whatever the treatment, the effect will depend on the experience and aptitude of the practitioner. It is crucial that the implants are correctly placed with great accuracy.

acupuncture, the gold implants, once inserted, are left in the body, making the effect permanent.

For the procedure, the animal is sedated and prepared for surgery. Under sterile conditions, small pieces of gold wire ('beads') are inserted through a large syringe, and permanently deposited at the selected acupuncture points. Several studies have documented the long-term beneficial effect of this technique in dogs suffering from arthritis of the hip. In my opinion, this treatment is best performed by a veterinary surgeon who is also a competent acupuncturist.

The origin of acupuncture

Acupuncture has been used in the treatment of both people and animals for thousands of years. Originally, acupuncture was merely one aspect of traditional Chinese medicine. Some vets today do use acupuncture in this way, analysing their patients according to the Chinese five-element-theory. Others use a more Western approach, focusing mainly on the pathological and anatomical aspects and, rather than conducting a full holistic analysis of the individual patient, selecting acupuncture points based primarily on what joint is affected.

Mode of action

According to the philosophy underlying traditional Chinese medicine, energy (chi) flows along channels in the body referred to as meridians. If the energy doesn't flow freely, the resulting stagnation leads to the development of disease. Acupuncture points are located on the meridians and can be stimulated to affect the flow of chi.

Using a traditional Chinese five-element analysis of the patient's symptoms (taking into account many factors, including an evaluation of the pulses and the appearance of the tongue), the traditional acupuncturist will analyse the case to understand the specific blockage of the chi and, on this basis, decide where to place the needles to allow the chi to flow freely and the patient to return to health.

Over the years, extensive scientific research has explored a more Western and, perhaps, modern explanation of the mode of action of acupuncture. Scientific Western research focuses on the field of neurophysiology and has found a correlation between the ancient, well-described acupuncture points, and areas in the body that contain a high concentration of blood vessels and nerve endings. Stimulation of these areas releases a range of transmitters, both in the area being treated and in the brain. This release of neurotransmitters, among them endorphins, works as a natural form of pain relief.

These two different explanations of how acupuncture works to relieve pain do not, strictly speaking, contradict each other. In many cases, the needles would no doubt end up being inserted at the same acupuncture points for the same patient. You might choose to see it as two different maps leading to the same place, or two different languages describing the same phenomenon.

ACUPUNCTURE SUMMARY

❖ Take your dog or cat to see a veterinary acupuncturist if they suffer from osteoarthritis
❖ Gold-bead implants can help achieve a lasting effect without the need for lifelong treatment
❖ There are different approaches to acupuncture

MANUAL THERAPIES

For the purposes of this book, I will use manipulative therapies, or manual therapies, as a collective term describing chiropractic, osteopathy, and cranio-sacral therapy, among others.

These treatment forms are all based on gentle physical manipulation of muscles, connective tissue, and joints. Although there are various approaches and schools of practice, these modalities are similar enough to be discussed together in this context.

For ease of reference, the term osteopathy is used here to apply also to other manipulative therapies, such as chiropractic and cranio-sacral therapy.

When to see an osteopath

The manual treatment forms are used primarily to support the musculoskeletal system of the body, correcting any problems involving muscles, connective tissue, bones or joints. Manual treatments can be extremely useful in a wide range of situations, ranging from the treatment of painful pathological conditions to prevention and support for the healthy, active dog.

The active lifestyle involved in hunting, agility and other dog activities – including plain rough-and-tumble play – can lead to a multitude of minor strains and injuries that can be relieved through osteopathy or massage. Manipulative treatments are not limited to the preservation of health and free movement, however, being equally useful in the treatment of serious conditions, such as in connection with rehabilitation after injury or surgery, or in the case of more chronic conditions, such as osteoarthritis. In all of these very different situations, manipulative therapies can make a major difference to the outcome, and help reduce the need for conventional pain relief.

In my opinion, one or other of the manipulative treatment forms is likely to help anyone who has a musculoskeletal problem. They can be used together with acupuncture, which is also indicated for most conditions that, simply put, affect the way the body moves.

Osteopathy around the world

Manual therapies in their varying forms are available all over the world. This is an area where most practitioners will probably not be veterinary surgeons, although many veterinary surgeons do have additional qualifications in chiropractic or osteopathy.

In many countries, regulations allow for this, provided the patient has been diagnosed by a vet and cleared for the particular therapy prior to treatment. Many veterinary nurses have extra qualifications in these fields. In some countries the law demands that a practitioner work under the direct supervision of a veterinary surgeon.

Increasingly, larger veterinary centres offer osteopathy and physiotherapy as part of the recommended aftercare of orthopaedic patients.

The osteopathic consultation

The practitioner uses her hands to gently manipulate the tissues, exploring and correcting the range of motion of affected joints and other structures. There is no pain, and excessive force is not involved. Indeed, the approach is often so natural and suggestive that it may seem as though the practitioner is just having a chat with the patient while feeling her way along their body, and not really doing anything at all!

There are no drugs, needles or other instruments involved in the treatment, and the sudden wrenching and crunching manipulations of the old-fashioned human chiropractor are not considered appropriate in the treatment of animals, and seem to have become rarer in any context.

Sometimes the practitioner will give instructions for exercises or massage techniques to be continued at home.

Duration of treatment

The need for repeated visits to your manipulative therapist will naturally depend on the character of the problem being treated. A single treatment may be enough to treat a minor acute injury. Peak performance dogs used for sport or hunting often benefit from regular adjustments – much like any other athlete.

During the recovery period following a more serious injury or an orthopaedic surgical procedure, your dog may require regular treatments and evaluations over several weeks or months. If your dog or cat has an ongoing chronic problem, such as osteoarthritis, lifelong regular manipulative therapy can increase their mobility and quality of life, while reducing the need for pain medication.

Mode of action

Any painful event will lead to an alteration of the gait, however temporary, as the body tries to spare the affected limb. This invariably leads to increased strain on other parts of the body as the flow of natural movement is disturbed. A gentle adjustment of the range and mode of movement can make a crucial difference in relieving these imbalances.

I have pooled together several different techniques in this section. In slightly different ways, they all strive to optimise the movement of the body by stimulating muscle, bone and nerves to shed inappropriate acquired patterns of movement.

OSTEOPATHY SUMMARY

❖ If your dog or cat suffers from a musculoskeletal problem, ask for a referral to an osteopath
❖ Manual therapy is crucial to aid recovery after injury or orthopaedic surgery
❖ As your dog or cat ages, look out for signs of stiffness, pain, or decreased mobility

BACH FLOWER REMEDIES

When to use Bach flower remedies

Bach flower remedies can be a first step in a wide range of situations where, without the presence of specific physical illness, extra support is required.

The treatment is always chosen on the basis of the emotional state of the patient alone: nothing else is considered. An indicated selection of remedies can provide invaluable support when dogs or cats have to travel, move house, accept a new addition to the household or cope with the stress of fireworks, thunderstorms or the absence of their main carers.

In cases of established behavioural problems, the flower remedies can be given to aid behavioural training, and in cases of physical illness they can supplement the treatment prescribed by your vet.

The idea behind Bach flower remedies

is that every imbalance will lead to an altered mental state. Disease of any kind will affect the individual's mood and behaviour. As is the case with the other holistic treatment methods, this is a system of medicine that was developed to treat humans, but which is equally suitable to animals.

Dr Bach to the rescue

Rescue Remedy is by far the best-known version of Dr Bach's flower remedies. The mixture consists of five flower remedies (impatiens, star-of-Bethlehem, cherry plum, rock rose and clematis). This mixture suits a common reaction to a situation of acute stress. It is the only available ready-to-use, pre-mixed treatment. Rescue Remedy can be put on a treat, added to drinking water or given directly into the mouth of the patient. It is important to give frequent doses for optimal effect.

Note: Bach's Rescue Remedy is also available as a pastille. This contains the artificial sweetener xylitol, which is toxic to dogs and cats and must be avoided (see page 30). Choose the liquid instead.

Bach flower remedies around the world

Bach flower remedies are available all over the world; the popular Rescue Remedy (sometimes called emergency essence) being the most readily available. For more specific treatment, you can buy a kit of all 38 flower remedies, or you can select and buy the individual flower remedies that you have decided are appropriate to treat your animal.

There is no difference in the application of flower remedies to animals and people. Others after Dr Bach have been inspired to develop their own series of remedies; one example of this being the Australian Bush Remedies.

The treatment: do-it-yourself

Dr Bach aimed to develop a very simple approach that, unlike homeopathy, consists of only a limited number of remedies that can be combined freely for easy home treatment. It was Bach's intention that (human) patients should be able to identify their own disorder, then select, make, and administer their own treatment as well as assess their own improvement. The whole point was to empower the individual and reject the notion that we need experts to tell us how we are and what will make us better.

Practitioners now undergo training in the use of Bach flower remedies, so, if you would like guidance in the selection of the most suitable remedies for yourself, it is possible in many countries to see a Bach flower therapist. The system was developed for home treatment, however, so don't hesitate to have a go, whether for yourself or your animal. As long as you don't neglect to take your pet to the vet if he is ill, and don't stop prescribed medications, you can do no harm.

You will find all you need to get going on the following pages of this book. Bach flower remedies were intended to be easy for anyone to apply – and they are.

Duration of treatment

If you are treating an acute episode of stress or supporting your animal through a brief stressful event, such as an evening of fireworks or a trip to the vet, a few doses during the course of a single day will probably be enough. In cases of more lasting and individual issues, it is important to keep up the treatment and give several daily doses.

It is my impression that Bach flower remedies, whether for people or animals, often do not achieve the desired effect simply because the dosing is not frequent enough or the treatment period is too short. Of course, a positive outcome always depends on the correct selection of remedies, but in most ongoing situations a few doses here and there (even of the perfect remedy or mix of remedies) will make little difference. Once you have made up your treatment bottle, remember to give at least four daily doses for several weeks until the problem has been resolved.

Having said that, it rarely makes sense to continue the same treatment for years. If you find that you have to keep using the flower remedies to maintain the effect, it may be worth considering a deeper-acting treatment to achieve a permanent cure.

What's what: Bach flower remedies and homeopathy

Although there are similarities, Bach flower remedies are not the same as homeopathy. The remedies are produced in an entirely different way. The two biggest differences in the application of the two forms of treatment are, firstly, that Bach flower remedies are always prescribed entirely on the basis of the patient's mood: physical symptoms are never considered. Secondly, whereas the homeopath has to select a single remedy from thousands to suit the patient on all levels, there are only 38 Bach flower remedies, from which the patient (or the patient's carer) is free to create a mixture to best reflect their emotional state. Bach flower remedies are truly designed to be simple and easy.

The medicine

Bach flower remedies are never chosen to treat physical symptoms or disease directly. The remedies are selected based only on the emotional state of the patient. This, together with the limited number of remedies, is why this system of treatment is so simple to use. Remember that, from its inception, the whole point was to provide a system of home treatment without the need for extensive study.

The only pre-made treatment bottle is Rescue Remedy, which suits a situation of acute stress (whether the stress is caused by an imminent exam, in the case of a human, a trip to the vet for a dog, or exposure to an evening of fireworks for a cat). For all situations other than short-term acute stress, the remedy or remedy mixture must be carefully selected for each individual.

Based on the descriptions of the 38 flower remedies on pages 114 and 115, simply select the remedy or remedies that best reflect the mood of the patient at the time of treatment. If a single remedy covers the patient's mood, use only the one; if more than one remedy applies to the individual to be treated, mix them together. If you end up selecting more than six or seven remedies, you probably need to sharpen your focus.

The treatment bottle

The only premixed combination contains rock rose, impatiens, cherry plum, star-of-Bethlehem and clematis. It is sold by various companies under different names, with Rescue Remedy, emergency essence and crisis remedy being well known the world over. This mixture treats situations of acute stress. It may be given after an accident and before and during stressful events, such as exams for humans or nail-clipping, vet visits, grooming, transport and the like for animals.

For more individual or long-term problems, you need to make up a selection that suits the patient.

To make an individualised treatment mix, first select the remedies you want to include. This can be done quickly and easily using the 38 remedy descriptions on page 114. Consider both the patient's personality and the symptoms of the heightened emotional state that you wish to treat.

From the remedy stock bottles of your selected remedies, simply add two drops of each remedy to your treatment bottle. A 30ml glass or plastic dropper bottle works perfectly as an individual treatment bottle. If you are keeping the treatment bottle in the fridge, just fill the bottle with spring water and add your drops to that.

It is helpful to keep the bottle with you, in which case adding a teaspoon of alcohol, such as brandy or vodka, to the mixture will preserve it without refrigeration. From this treatment bottle, give four drops at least four times daily.

Another method, more suited to short-term treatment or situations where one remedy is all you need (when you may not want to bother making a treatment bottle), is to give two drops directly from the stock bottle, either dissolved in water or directly into the patient's mouth. There is no difference in effect between the two methods (taking two drops from the stock bottle or four drops from the treatment bottle).

Using the stock bottle just uses up the remedy faster, and is not very convenient if you are giving several remedies several times a day.

Taking the medicine

Bach flower remedies, unlike homeopathic remedies, can be given in food or drink. If you are treating your dog or cat, the simplest method is to put the dose on a small treat. This means that, even with frequent dosing, your animal won't mind at all. In all but the most acute situations, Bach flower remedies work best when given several times a day for several weeks or months.

Storing the medicine

Bach flower remedies are not sensitive to smell and temperature in the way that homeopathic remedies are. The stock bottles will keep for years at room temperature. The treatment bottle will be fine for many weeks if kept in the fridge, or if a little alcohol is added to the bottle.

Making the medicine

Bach sourced all his remedies from the British countryside. Apart from one (water from a local spring), they are all made from wild plants. The flower remedies are produced either by the sun method, in which the flowers soak in water in full sunlight for three hours, or, when the remedy is not made from a flower, by boiling the plant material for 30 minutes.

When the energy or essence of the plant has been transferred to the water by one of these methods, the 'activated' water is diluted with an equal amount of brandy to make up the mother tincture. This is later diluted further to make up the stock bottles that you can buy, either individually or in a kit containing all 38 flower essences.

It was Dr Bach's intention that anyone should be able to produce their own flower remedies, and if you feel so inclined and have the botanical knowledge to find the source material, there is nothing to stop you doing this. More commonly, you can buy the stock bottles and make up your own treatment bottle as described above.

The origin of Bach flower remedies

Dr Edward Bach was a British medical doctor who spent a large part of his career doing research on the importance of the microorganisms of the intestines, and their relationship to health. Today, the microbiome is a big buzzword in medical research, but Dr Bach, visionary that he was, chose this as his field of interest a hundred years ago. He was also intimately familiar with homeopathy: at one point working alongside the doctors at the Homeopathic Hospital in London.

Inspired by homeopathy and the results that the homeopathic doctors were achieving, Dr Bach held two main convictions that led him to pursue a different route, and ultimately to leave London and the medical establishment of the time to develop his own system of medicine.

1

FEAR

Rock rose (for emergencies and total panic, as may be felt during fireworks. Terror)

Mimulus (fear of certain everyday things, such as darkness, noise, or being home alone)

Cherry plum (sensitivity, nervousness and hysteria leading to lack of control. Biting)

Aspen (vague, unexplainable fears. General nervousness without clear cause)

Red chestnut (exaggerated concern and worry for others)

2

UNCERTAINTY
Cerato (overly dependent on others, lacking confidence)

Scleranthus (indecisive, changeable, quietly unstable)

Gentian (easily discouraged. Gives up at the slightest difficulty)

Gorse (hopelessness. Has given up)

Hornbeam (feeling weak and unable to cope. Tired)

Wild oat (lack of focus. Easily distracted, frustrated, restless)

3

INSUFFICIENT INTEREST IN PRESENT CIRCUMSTANCES
Clematis (drowsy and unenthusiastic)

Honeysuckle (living in the past. Missing old home, carer or companion)

Wild rose (apathetic, never standing up for oneself, resigned)

Olive (worn out from suffering or abuse. Tired after a great effort)

White chestnut (constant worry. Inability to let go)

Mustard (sad and depressed without obvious reason. Can't be cheered up)

Chestnut bud (slow to learn. Repeats the same mistakes)

4

LONELINESS
Water violet (calm and quiet individuals who keep to themselves. Reserved, isolated)

Impatiens (spontaneous and impatient. Restless)

Heather (open and communicative. Self-centred. Hates being alone)

OVERSENSITIVE TO INFLUENCES

Agrimony (cheerful and sociable. Appears friendly and happy. Gives in to avoid conflict)

Centaury (over-anxious to please. Can't stand up for himself)

Walnut (change and transition. May be led astray by others or dominated)

Holly (jealousy, envy. Suspicious. Territorial. Aggressive)

DESPONDENCY OR DESPAIR

Larch (lack of confidence. So convinced they will fail that they don't even try)

Pine (extreme pleaser, blames himself even when someone else has failed. Guilt)

Elm (responsible and hardworking, but may be overwhelmed if too much is asked of them)

Sweet chestnut (hopelessness. Lacks the strength to go on. Intense grief)

Star-of-Bethlehem (aftereffects of shock. Distressed, but unable to accept consolation)

Willow (bitter and insulted. Self-pity and resentment)

Oak (keeps going in spite of great pain or adversity. Reliable. Stoical)

Crab apple (cleansing. Feeling of having to wash away a stain. Over-grooming)

OVER-CARE FOR THE WELFARE OF OTHERS

Chicory (possessive, manipulative. Corrects others. Demands attention. Dislikes being alone)

Vervain (strong willed, domineering, doesn't give up. Overenthusiastic)

Vine (confident, domineering)

Beech (irritable, intolerant, hard on others, aggressive)

Rock water (competitive, confident, inflexible, rigid. Likes routine)

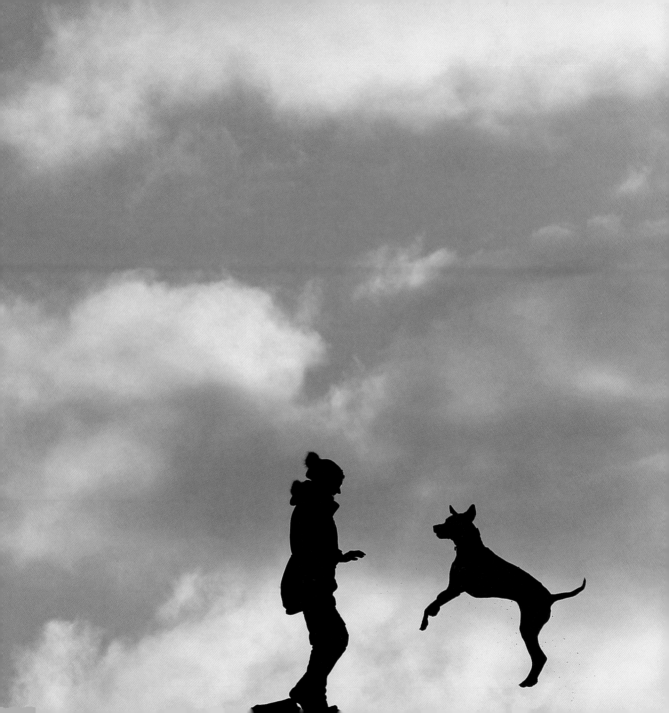

Firstly, he firmly believed in the value of leaving patients in charge of their own health. As a doctor, he found it intrinsically wrong that we become so out of touch with ourselves that we need a doctor to tell us the state of our health, and what treatments to take, and then later, return to the doctor's office to be told if the treatments worked, unable, apparently, to tell for ourselves.

Dr Bach felt that each of us should strive to know our own state of health, and be able to act to improve it when needed. He wanted to take the expert out of the equation and empower individuals to take charge of their own health, and their own treatment.

Secondly, he believed that any imbalance in the body, even serious physical illness, originates in the mind. The mental state reflects the state of health, and any physical disease will be the result of an imbalance that will be reflected in the mental state.

In 1930, Dr Bach left his medical practice in London to retreat to his home in Oxfordshire, where he spent the last six years of his life developing this simple do-it-yourself system to treat any mental state, and therefore, according to him, any imbalance and subsequent illness. All 38 remedies (37 of which are plant material) were found locally in the countryside surrounding his home.

Dr Bach's house in Oxfordshire, Mount Vernon, is owned by the Dr Bach Healing Trust, and is open to visitors.

Mode of action

Dr Bach said that his remedies freed the mind, bringing clarity and self-healing. He compared this to the healing effect of music or nature. No scientific explanation has yet been established.

Bach's seven reactions and 38 remedies

Dr Bach organised his 38 flower remedies under seven headings representing seven fundamental emotional states. In each of the seven categories, the flower remedies represent different aspects of the basic emotional state, as listed in the table overleaf.

BACH'S FLOWER REMEDY SUMMARY

❖ Bach flower remedies are different from homeopathy and from herbal medicine
❖ Bach flower remedies are particularly suitable for home treatment
❖ The remedies are selected entirely on the basis of the patient's emotional state

HOMEOPATHY

When to see a homeopath

Any condition can benefit from homeopathic treatment. Homeopathy has a marked effect on the immune system, and is absolutely ideal for treating immune imbalances such as autoimmune disease and allergies. Whether the allergy affects the digestion, the airways or the skin (causing chronic recurring diarrhoea, asthma or allergic skin disease), homeopathy is, in my opinion, the treatment of choice. If you know someone who suffers from allergy in any form, call a homeopath. If that someone is a cat or dog, call a homeopathic vet.

I also find homeopathy to be especially helpful when treating hormonal imbalances (eg infertility or false pregnancy), and metabolic disease (thyroid disease and Cushing's disease).

Homeopathy around the world

With the notable exception of a few Scandinavian countries, homeopathy is widely available and well known around the world, and in many places, homeopathic treatment for humans is an integral part of the public healthcare system. In England, the London Homeopathic hospital was opened in 1849, and, together with four other homeopathic hospitals, was included in the British National Health Service from its inception immediately after World War II. Sadly, recent cutbacks in the UK have limited the public's access to free homeopathic healthcare, whereas, in Switzerland, homeopathy was added to the publicly funded healthcare system as recently as 2012.

Homeopathy has been used to treat people for 230 years, and in the past 40 years or so an increasing number of vets all over the world have begun practising homeopathy for both companion and farm animals. Note that, in many countries, only vets can legally use homeopathy to treat animals. Page 215 explains where to find vets with post-graduate qualifications in homeopathy.

The homeopathic consultation

Regardless of whether the patient is a human, a dog or a cat, the effect of the homeopathic treatment is entirely dependent on the patient getting the correct remedy. As described in the introduction to this chapter, the remedy will never be selected on the basis of a disease diagnosis alone. The remedy has to fit the individual patient, taking all their symptoms into account. Ten patients with the exact same diagnosis can be expected to find a cure from ten different remedies. As there are thousands of remedies for the homeopath to choose from, making the all-important match between each patient and their correct remedy is a challenge that requires experience and time.

Most homeopathic vets spend an hour or more with a new patient, examining them, observing them and, most of all, asking the people who care for them about the animal's character, preferences, life history, and so on. Only when a full picture emerges will the homeopath be able to select the remedy that best suits the patient. Most carers enjoy the hour-long conversation and the chance to share all their experiences of their companion animal in health and disease, while most dogs and cats relax (even those who generally find visits to the veterinary clinic very stressful),

as they are mostly left to explore the room and interact as they please under the ever-observant eye of the homeopath.

Duration of treatment

Homeopathic treatment is rarely expected to be ongoing, although there are exceptions. I have, for instance, treated dogs and cats with severe arthritis or irreversible liver or kidney damage. Ongoing homeopathic treatment (over several years) was needed to keep these patients free of symptoms; because the organ damage was irreparable, a complete cure was never going to be possible.

However, in the majority of cases, even in serious and chronic disease, the aim of treatment will be to effect a change that lasts, even after the treatment is stopped. After all, to be considered cured, the patient must require no further treatment of any kind – and this is certainly the rule.

In my homeopathic clinic, I typically see a chronically ill patient for a monthly follow-up until they are well. For some, this amounts to only two or three visits; for others, it requires monthly visits for half a year or more to find the right remedy and see the full effect of treatment. The individual approach makes it hard to predict each course of treatment, but, when new carers inquire prior to treatment, my general advice is to be prepared to come at least three times over as many months. In my clinic, I set aside one hour for the first consultation, and half-an-hour for follow-up visits. It is generally not a good idea to start other new treatments at the same time as starting homeopathy. Always remember to consult your homeopathic vet if you are considering immunotherapy, acupuncture, new supplements or any other changes alongside the homeopathic treatment. This includes routine parasite control and vaccinations.

If your animal is being treated for acute disease, such as uncomplicated acute diarrhoea or maybe a case of kennel cough, the situation is very different, and you should expect to see an almost immediate effect. In these cases, one or two visits should suffice.

Homeopathic medicine

Homeopathic medicines, often referred to as homeopathic remedies, are produced at homeopathic pharmacies according to a specific method of serial dilutions. Most homeopathic medicines are made from plants or minerals, but there are also remedies made from a wide range of other sources, such as animal materials, pharmaceuticals, and everything else under the sun. Whatever the source of the remedy, it is the specific method of serial dilution, together with the manner in which it is prescribed, that makes a medicine homeopathic.

The remedy comes in many forms, from liquid to powders; pills and tablets. There is absolutely no therapeutic difference. The choice of tablets or drops is entirely a matter of personal preference and ease of administration. Each remedy will be available in all forms and in a full range of strengths (referred to as potencies). The exact same medicines are used for humans and animals. Actually, I quite enjoy the fact that, in homeopathy, we treat animals using medicines tested on humans.

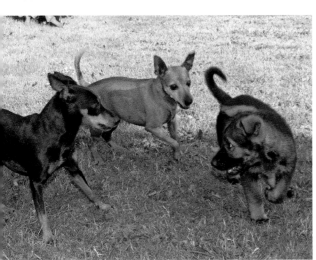

In most countries, homeopathic remedies are freely available and do not require a prescription.

You may get the remedy from your homeopathic vet at the time of the consultation, or they may simply advise you on which remedy to buy. Homeopathic medicine is inexpensive; the costly part of the treatment is the time and expertise involved in choosing the correct remedy. Many health-food shops carry a range of homeopathic remedies, and most large homeopathic pharmacies sell medicines online. This means that, no matter where you live, getting hold of homeopathic medicine should not be a problem. See page 216 for a list of pharmacies.

Understanding potencies

When the remedy is made through a 1/100 dilution at each step, we talk of the C scale, and the different strengths or potencies are 6C, 30C, 200C, and so on. When, as is more common in some countries, remedies are produced through a series of 1/10 dilutions, we refer to the D or X scale, and to the potencies as D6, D30 and D200 or 6X, 30X and 200X.

Even though the C-scale remedies will be much more dilute than those in the D or X scale, it is the number of dilution steps rather than the concentration itself that determines the medicinal power. For all practical purposes, this means that the scale (the letter) can be ignored. A remedy in the potency D30 can be used exactly as the same remedy in the potency 30C. Potency selection is for the professional homeopath.

For home treatments, 30 (whether C, D or X) is a nice, middle-strength, all-round potency to use.

How to give a remedy to your cat or dog

Even dogs and cats who are notoriously averse to accepting pills generally happily take homeopathic medicine. Administration is made very easy by the fact that the remedy has no bad flavour, and does not need to be swallowed. The key to success is to remember that homeopathic medicine is absorbed through contact with the mucous membrane of the mouth. This means that the second the medicine touches the inside of the mouth (the tongue, the gums or the inside of the cheek), the dose has been absorbed. There is no need to make the patient hold the medicine in the mouth or, indeed, swallow it. They may, of course, suck on it or swallow it if they like, but, as soon as the medicine is in the mouth, the dose is given, and what happens to it next is unimportant. If the pill or tablet ends up on the floor after one second in the mouth, that is fine, too.

Remember to always give homeopathic medicine away from food, with no food allowed for at least ten minutes before and after the dose. Give no treats for taking the medicine; indeed, the medicine (at least in pill form) tastes like sugar and is a treat in itself.

It is okay to touch the remedy, provided you don't clutch a pill in a sweaty hand for too long. A dry hand is absolutely fine for handling the medicine and swiftly placing it in the corner of the animal's mouth. For large dogs, often the easiest approach is simply to pull down the lip and put a pill in the corner of the mouth or on the gums when your dog is resting – more often than not, your dog won't even wake up.

A dose is a dose

It's not possible to give too much or too little in each dose, so don't worry about the amount. It is, of course, important that the remedy is correct, and that the potency is well chosen, but how many drops or pills are given in a single dose is of no importance. The dose is a signal – a message or an energetic input, if you like. Any amount will transfer the signal.

This means that you can intensify the treatment by giving two daily doses instead of one, but not by doubling the amount in a single dose, as this will make no difference at all.

Similarly, the size of the dose bears no relation to the size of the patient.

A dose is indeed a dose, and a pill or two will do the job, whether the patient is a mouse, an elephant, a tiny kitten or an adult Saint Bernard.

Giving a homeopathic remedy to a dog or a cat

Homeopathic medicine must always be given directly into the mouth and away from food. The remedy may be swallowed, although it is not absorbed in the stomach but rather from direct contact with the mucous membrane of the mouth before it even has a chance to reach the stomach. What this means, in practice, is that as soon as the medicine is in the mouth, you can ignore what happens to it. Just pop it in. Nothing could be easier.

How to store homeopathic medicine

Homeopathic medicine in pill or tablet form never goes off: remedies have been known to remain active after more than two hundred years. Liquid remedy is a watery solution, so it will decay, sometimes as soon as a few weeks after opening.

While time alone will have no detrimental effect on homeopathic pills, they can be antidoted and lose all medicinal properties. The two main things to avoid are extreme temperatures and strong smells. Homeopathic remedies are sensitive to both cold and heat. In practice, this just means that they will not work if exposed to a temperature below 0 degrees Celsius, and that you should avoid leaving remedies exposed to sunlight. Never leave remedies in the car, which may get very hot if parked in the sun. Room temperature is ideal.

Don't leave your medicine on top of a microwave or computer. I used to be very worried about even having a computer in the same room as my homeopathic remedies, but all of today's wireless networks don't seem to reduce the effect of homeopathic medicines.

Strong-smelling substances are the other main thing to look out for. Don't store your medicine next to perfumes, scented candles, aromatic oils, incense, camphor ointment, and the like. Ideally, keep your dog or cat away from these substances altogether when they are receiving homeopathic treatment. As long as these precautions are taken, you can keep using your remedies long after the obligatory expiration date.

Side effects

Homeopathic medicine has no side effects and can never do harm. The worst that can possibly happen is that the remedy doesn't resonate with the patient, in which case it will have no effect at all.

This makes it quite safe for you to experiment with treating minor ailments yourself: the worst that can happen is that you give the wrong remedy, which means it will have no effect. As long as you always have your animal checked by a vet to make sure you don't overlook a potentially serious condition, and as long as you don't stop giving prescribed medications without consulting your vet, you really can do no harm.

No strong-smelling products: inside or out

Strong-smelling substances can antidote homeopathic medicine. Avoid giving your animal garlic in any form. Whether for internal or external use, strong smells such as garlic, peppermint, essential oils and the like, must be avoided. Increasingly, natural flea and tick products as well as herbal supplements include these ingredients, so make sure to check the labels, ask your homeopathic vet, or simply avoid the product if you are in doubt.

Serious or chronic illness will require an experienced homeopath, of course. Cancer, epilepsy and autoimmune disease are not appropriate cases for home treatment. Even a fully qualified medical doctor or veterinary surgeon undertakes a further three to four years of study to become a competent homeopath. Seek professional help if your animal is seriously ill.

However, if you feel like getting your feet wet and you want to try a remedy to treat situations such as uncomplicated acute diarrhoea, kennel cough or car sickness, you will do no harm. Don't become disillusioned, however, if your remedy doesn't work. Try again or take your cat or dog to see a professional.

See the section on page 123 for more information on using homeopathy at home, and page 215 on finding a veterinary homeopath.

Aggravations

Sometimes, the initial reaction to a homeopathic remedy will be a marked worsening of the symptoms. This is not a side effect but rather a very positive sign that the remedy has hit the mark and that healing has begun. It is not necessary to experience aggravations for healing to occur, and most patients don't. If they do happen, however, it is confirmation that the remedy is correct, and a promising sign that improvement is on the way.

An aggravation will never hurt the patient: the worst that can happen as a result of homeopathic treatment is absolutely nothing. This will be the case when the remedy was wrong and the homeopath must come up with a better prescription. It is not unusual for the second or even third remedy to be the one that works. Picking the one correct remedy among thousands is no easy task. As they say: the more I practice, the luckier I get. The more experienced the homeopath, the more likely that she will be able to identify the correct remedy to cure each patient at the first attempt.

Homeopathy in name only

The ever-important holistic principle of individualised treatment is absolutely fundamental to the effect of homeopathic remedies. In fact, what makes a treatment homeopathic is not the prescription of homeopathic medicines, but the fact that the remedy is selected according to homeopathic principles: meaning that it must very closely match the patient according to well-defined criteria. Each patient needs their exact matching remedy.

In contrast to this, conventional medicines are given based on the problem (disease diagnosis) alone. The advantage of the latter approach is easy to spot: giving a medicine based on a diagnosis is a 'one-size-fits-all' approach. It is quick, easy, and cheap.

It is hardly surprising, then, that the temptation to simplify homeopathic treatments is strong. Walk into a health-food shop in most countries in the world and you will find the shelves stocked with 'homeopathic cough medicine,' 'homeopathic sleeping medicine,' and the like. Perhaps from an altruistic desire to make homeopathy more easily available, perhaps lured by the chance of easy profit, poly-pharmacy simplifies the time-consuming aspects of individual prescribing by applying a reductionist approach to homeopathic treatment. It is, in short, a doomed attempt to square the circle by using homeopathic medicine in a conventional way: a product to fit a condition.

Poly-pharmacy (using remedy mixtures containing anywhere from a few to more than a hundred homeopathic remedies) seems to work on the principle that, if you don't know what remedy the patient needs, you simply mix a load of remedies together and hope to get lucky. Some patients will experience some degree of relief from such products, but many

more will not – and it will never remotely equal the potential of a single well-chosen remedy. In their defence, these mixtures don't harm anyone (because homeopathic medicine has no side effects), but neither do they do much good. Worst of all, they give homeopathy a bad name, as too many patients will have negative experiences, and then say that they tried homeopathy and it didn't work.

Kinesiology and vega-testing are other examples of cutting corners in an attempt to make homeopathy easier and less time-consuming, as the practitioner needs no homeopathic training and doesn't have to be familiar with the properties of homeopathic medicines. This undermining of such a powerful treatment modality is a constant source of frustration. The wrong remedy will do nothing at all, while the right remedy has the potential to cure even the most serious condition. Time and effort spent finding the right homeopathic treatment is rarely wasted.

The origin of homeopathy

Homeopathy is based on ancient principles described as early as the Greek philosophers, more than 2000 years ago. The German doctor Samuel Hahnemann developed the medical practice of homeopathy in the late 1700s, and is regarded as the father of homeopathy. He formulated the ruling principle of similia similibus curentur ('like cures like'), which states that a substance that can produce symptoms in a healthy individual will cure the same symptoms when they appear in a sick individual.

The past 200 years have contributed a wealth of clinical experience, and more remedies are being introduced all the time. There are currently close to 5000 available homeopathic remedies.

Mode of action

The process of producing homeopathic medicines involves a series of dilutions,

It depends ...

Questions such as 'What homeopathic remedy should I give a dog with allergic eczema?' or 'What is a good homeopathic remedy for … ?' can only ever be answered correctly by someone who understands the principles of homeopathy, with the oft-repeated and probably frustrating answer, 'That depends entirely on what remedy suits the particular patient.'

according to Hahnemann's specific instructions, to beyond the point at which a chemical analysis of the remedy would be able to detect any trace of the original substance. The fact that there is often not a single molecule of the original material present in the remedy has for more than two centuries puzzled everyone trying to understand the mode of action of homeopathic medicines.

'How can it work when there is nothing in it?' has been the question. An answer has emerged in the 21st century as the focus has shifted from a chemical perspective to the point of view of physics. Led by the Nobel Prize-winning French scientist Dr Luc Montagnier, scientists are now demonstrating the emission of electromagnetic resonance from highly potentised (ie very dilute) homeopathic remedies.

Homeopathy at home

Homeopathy is invaluable in treating common acute ailments in animals and humans alike.

If you would like to try a homeopathic remedy on your dog or cat (or maybe on yourself), go ahead: it really can't hurt. The following pages contain some guidelines and pointers to increase your chance of success.

If you are treating an acute condition, you can repeat a dose every hour or two. In acute situations, the effect will generally be immediate but may not be long-lived. The rule

is always to repeat when the effect wanes.

If you are treating a chronic condition, give a daily dose for a week to a dog or cat. If you are taking a remedy yourself that you feel fits you at a deep (constitutional) level, take only a single dose. Clinical experience shows that dogs and cats (with their shorter lifespans, higher body temperature, and faster heart and respiration rates) use up a homeopathic dose faster, so therefore often need longer courses than humans. A good rule of thumb is that if you see no effect at all after six doses, it is probably the wrong remedy and nothing is going to happen. This means that, in an acute situation, the remedy should work within a day. If it doesn't, stop and reconsider your choice of remedy. In a chronic condition, don't give your chosen remedy for more than a week. Remember that chronic conditions are more difficult to treat and more likely to require professional guidance.

An ideal potency for home treatment is 30C (or D30 or 30X). Giving a homeopathic remedy can never hurt your animal. However, the effect of your treatment naturally depends on your ability to pinpoint the correct remedy. The more you know about homeopathy, and the more homeopathic remedies you are familiar with, the higher the chance of success. It goes without saying that any sick

Code—breaker

A chemical analysis of a music CD would identify only polycarbonate plastic with traces of aluminium, and would be unable to say whether the CD was a recording of Beethoven or the Beatles. Similarly, chemical analysis of homeopathic remedies reveals only the base of water and alcohol, lactose or sucrose, depending on the chosen remedy form. Only when we look at the remedy from a physicist's point of view can the medicinal properties be decoded.

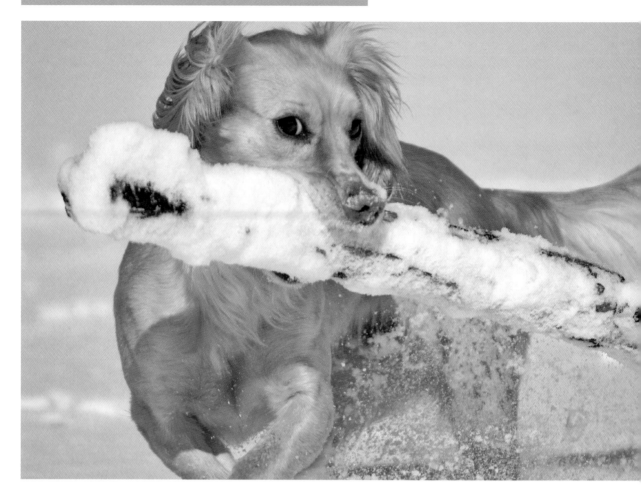

animal should be examined and diagnosed by a veterinary surgeon. Likewise, never stop prescribed medications without first discussing this with your veterinary surgeon.

With these precautions in mind, don't be afraid to experiment.

Levels of treatment

It is beyond the scope of this book to discuss the considerations of a professional veterinary homeopath when planning the treatment for an individual case. It takes three to four years of homeopathic study, and a lifetime of experience for a vet to learn how to use homeopathy to treat chronic illness such as allergies or epilepsy. However, rest assured that you can do no harm by having a go.

Generally speaking, chronic illness is treated at a constitutional level, meaning that all the characteristic traits of the patient have to be matched in the remedy selection. Treating acute illness is easier, as the remedy primarily has to match the symptoms of the acute disease.

The homeopathic principle is always to match the symptom picture of the patient to the symptom picture of the remedy. *Symptom* in this context covers all aspects, from appetite and thirst to behavioural traits, and so on. If there is a cough, what type of cough? What brings it on? What relieves it? If there is diarrhoea, what are the characteristic features?

The homeopathic remedy will cure

when it fits the patient like a glove fits a hand. Note that it is easy to become confused as to whether a description is about a patient or a medicine. This is simply because they have to be identical. The remedy must be chosen to reflect the patient. If the patient's symptom picture is like this, this medicine will fit.

The homeopath knows the remedies intimately and, when meeting a patient, always attempts to identify which remedy best fits the particular patient. There are thousands of remedies to choose from, but some are more commonly indicated than others.

In the following section, some of the most common remedies are described. Some of these are used mostly in deep-acting, constitutional treatment for chronic ailments, where the remedy must fit all aspects of the patient perfectly. Others are used primarily in the treatment of acute conditions, or on the basis of a strong tissue affinity combined with a specific symptom picture.

You may see a description that you recognize and decide to try the remedy. You may also choose simply to see this section as an illustration of the principles of homeopathic practice, and of the broad range of conditions that can be treated successfully with homeopathy – when the remedy fits the patient.

A short introduction to some common homeopathic remedies
Calcarea carbonica
Calc carb is an uncomplicated, 'earthy' personality type. Individuals belonging to this type, regardless of whether they are humans, dogs, cats, chickens or elephants, will share some common traits.

They particularly enjoy physical comforts: a Calc carb dog will certainly love his food and a comfortable place to relax in the sun or by the fire. They tend to be quite content with a fairly sedentary lifestyle. Calc carb types are often of a heavy build, and may

tend to put on weight easily; I find that this holds true especially for Calc carb cats. Calc carb individuals are by nature phlegmatic and easy-going, but may have a stubborn streak. A Calc carb dog may, for instance, sit down halfway through a walk, and simply refuse to move if your chosen route doesn't suit him.

Sometimes their hearty appetites extend to eating earth, sticks or even excrement. A Calc carb individual can, of course, fall ill with any number of ailments, but they seem to have a particular tendency to suffer from skeletal problems, such as dysplasia and osteoarthritis. An underactive thyroid is another common complaint among Calc carb individuals.

Calcarea phosphorica
Whereas Calc carb, as described above, is often heavy and calm to the point of maybe being considered lazy, Calc phos, on the other hand, is a lean, restless and active type that could never be accused of laziness.

This remedy suits many young dogs at an age when they seem to consist of nothing but long limbs and boundless energy, often testing the carer's patience with their constant desire for attention and activity. They are easily bored and, teenagers that they are, their desire for action may get them into trouble.

A Calc phos individual will often be hungry – indeed, they may be constantly eating or looking for food – but they will not put on weight, retaining instead their characteristic lean appearance.

When the type fits, Calc phos is often a good support remedy when growing pains cause lameness in active young dogs.

Natrum muriaticum
Nat mur is a sensitive, introverted and reserved personality type. They are generally quiet and keep to themselves, but may lash out in anger, especially if their personal boundaries are not respected. The Nat mur

cat may not allow himself to be picked up, and the Nat mur dog may not want to be petted by strangers in the street, or take kindly to being disturbed when he has retired to a quiet, private space in the house. Nat mur dogs and cats often ignore guests, or even leave the room to avoid contact with strangers, not being flirty, social types at all. They often form strong bonds with their carers, and may enjoy being stroked or cuddling on a lap; albeit 'on their terms.'

Their fundamentally private nature can be observed in various ways: some Nat mur individuals are very private about their toilet habits; others don't like direct eye contact. Being 'loners' by nature, Nat mur individuals tend to forge few but very deep and strong relationships in their lifetimes. If these bonds are broken, they can suffer greatly. Rehomed Nat mur animals often carry this trauma to the detriment of their health and wellbeing until the remedy helps them recover.

Nat mur individuals are generally quite sensitive to heat, and will not be hugging the fire or sunbathing, preferring instead a cooler spot. The cat who forgoes the radiator bed or the warm, sunny patch on the carpet, choosing instead to lie on a shady kitchen countertop or other cool surface, often responds well to Nat mur when the personality type fits. Another strong pointer to this remedy is that individuals will always be quite thirsty.

A Nat mur animal may, of course, suffer from almost any condition, but they do have a strong tendency toward skin problems. Many Nat mur cats develop urinary (especially kidney) problems, or an overactive thyroid.

Phosphorus

Phos is a spontaneous, enthusiastic, sociable and very extroverted personality type. Where the Nat mur types are very protective of their personal boundaries, it can almost seem as though Phos individuals do not have personal boundaries. They tend to be immediately friendly, seeing any stranger as their new best friend. This is the dog who happily follows someone home from the park, or the cat who sits on the front step and greets all who pass.

Phos individuals are thirsty. They tend to be slim and are often described as fast, athletic, and graceful in their movements. This is the cat who climbs nimbly to the top shelf, and the dog who strangers stop to admire – just to look at him go. They are so deeply sociable that being alone may be a problem for them. They thrive when they are part (or preferably the centre of) a group.

Phos is a sensitive type; sensitive to moods and atmosphere, and disliking raised voices. Some Phos animals even know when their carers fall ill before anyone else is aware of it.

This combination of sensitivity and lack of boundaries can make some Phos types quite fearful: sudden noises, thunderstorms, and being abandoned are common fears among these individuals. You may hear Phos described as a 'remedy for fear of fireworks.' This is only a partial truth. According to the previously described fundamental principles of homeopathy, the remedy will work only when it fits the individual patient. Therefore, it will help some dogs and cats who suffer from fear of fireworks (ie the Phos types), and there is certainly likely to be a relatively high proportion of Phos constitutional types among animals who are terrified of loud noises.

Apart from noise sensitivity and fear of being home alone, Phos individuals are predisposed toward colitis and asthma, although, of course, they may suffer from any physical problem.

Pulsatilla

Pulsatilla is a gentle and sweet type. Soft, loving and yielding, they will avoid conflict and generally aim to please. Their thirst is below average. Whether the Pulsatilla type is a child, a dog or a cat, their carers will often worry that they 'don't drink enough,' and some try to entice them to increase their fluid intake by adding water to their food. From the point of view of the homeopath, there is no ideal amount of water an individual should drink; rather, the presence or absence of thirst can be a very useful pointer or confirmatory symptom in the selection of the right remedy. Pulsatillas just don't feel thirsty.

They may be quite warm-blooded and avoid hot, stuffy rooms and direct sources of heat, or they may actively enjoy sunbathing or lying by the fire for a short period. They will always be quite quick to overheat and move away, perhaps to return once they have cooled down. Similarly, they are generally keen on endless hugs and kisses from their family, and can lie on the lap for hours (except when they get too hot and need to cool down).

Pulsatillas like everybody, as long as they are nice, but compared to a type like Phosphorus, who is right in your face, even if you have never met before, Pulsatillas can be a little shy at first, and need time to check out strangers to ensure they are indeed safe and gentle. Once reassured, they will be happy to make friends.

If they meet another dog or, indeed, a human whose body language doesn't reassure them, they will either lie down submissively or shy away. Often, they will come to their carers for support if faced with a potentially threatening situation. 'Love me and look after me' is what most Pulsatillas ask of others. Some Pulsatillas are specifically attracted to babies, and sometimes insist on going straight up to all children in the street; will seek out people with prams or strollers, and sometimes the affection is aimed at puppies rather than human youngsters.

There are certainly Pulsatilla males (these will be mild and gentle; almost feminine types), but Pulsatilla is primarily seen as a female remedy. The mothering instinct can be very strong, and, if allowed to breed, they will be excellent mothers, with endless patience and an equally endless milk supply. Pulsatilla has a strong affinity to the female hormonal system, and there will generally be some evidence of this in the Pulsatilla constitutional type.

Perhaps the problem belongs to the reproductive organs, or perhaps the symptoms started in (or are exacerbated during) oestrus. When the picture fits, Pulsatilla is often indicated in dogs with strong symptoms of false pregnancy.

Sepia

Sepia is sometimes described as an older, tougher, and more assertive Pulsatilla. There are certainly similarities. They are both predominantly female remedies, and both have a great affinity with the female reproductive system.

Sepia is by nature much chillier than Pulsatilla, and will happily lie in the sun or by the radiator for hours without overheating. They tend to have a sharper temperament and may, for instance, lash out aggressively at other dogs (especially other female dogs) much more readily than the sweet and yielding Pulsatilla is ever likely to do.

Sepia, like Pulsatilla, can be indicated when treating dogs suffering from false pregnancy. It is also helpful in many cases of urinary incontinence in bitches after neutering. In fact, any condition arising from pregnancy, birth, abortion, womb infections or neutering may be an indication for Sepia if the whole picture fits.

Nux vomica

Nux vomica is (like Sulphur) often used as a detox remedy. People commonly use it after over-indulging, and it has a great reputation as a first-aid remedy for indigestion as well as for hangovers. Animals can benefit from this approach when recovering from other types of poisoning.

When Nux vom is used on a deeper-acting, constitutional level, it fits a domineering personality who knows what he wants and is not afraid to go and get it. They may be very competitive and bossy.

Nux vom is a chilly type who enjoys soaking up heat from a fire, radiator or the sun. Their main affinity is with digestion. They tend to suffer some degree of indigestion, and many Nux vom types suffer from bloatedness or constipation. The liver is a sensitive organ in these individuals.

Lycopodium

Like Nux vomica, Lycopodium is a type that tends to suffer from indigestion. Also like Nux vom types, they often act in an assertive, if not even openly aggressive, manner.

However, Lycopodiums, unlike Nux vom, don't feel as confident as the image they project. Inside, they feel small and vulnerable, and will generally back down to avoid a fight if the focus of their anger turns out to be stronger than expected.

Arsenicum album

Individuals of the Arsenicum album type will always be very sensitive to cold. They hug the fire and can never get warm enough. I know both dogs and cats of this type who have actually caught fire, so keen were they to enjoy the full benefit of an open fireplace.

They are always thirsty animals, though typically drink only a little at a time, coming back frequently for another sip.

Arsenicum types are sensitive and vulnerable individuals who can be quite nervous and may even lash out if they feel threatened and cornered. They tend to be quite fastidious; keenly aware of a twig stuck in their coat, and going out of their way to avoid stepping in a muddy puddle. Their digestion is particularly sensitive, and they have a strong tendency to diarrhoea.

This remedy is used frequently and applied on many different levels. Anyone may benefit from Arsen alb at an acute level for a case of diarrhoea, whether viral or caused by food poisoning, when the symptoms fit the Arsen alb picture of vomiting, watery diarrhoea, prostration, weakness, thirsty for small sips of water, and shivering with cold.

Arsenicum is also an important remedy in the treatment of cancer and other life-threatening diseases. Many animals and humans have benefited from this remedy at the final stage of life.

In terms of chronic disease, Arsen alb individuals often suffer from problems of the digestive tract, airways or skin.

Staphysagria

Staphysagria is often a quiet and gentle individual, but also an unusually sensitive and vulnerable one. Somehow, they often become the ones everybody picks on – the born scapegoats, you might say. Whether they are actually being unfairly treated or merely perceive this to be the case, they are certainly quick to feel hurt or offended.

A typical example would be the cat who, when the family goes on holiday, urinates or defecates inappropriately. The perceived insult can also be a boyfriend moving in, causing the cat to urinate on his belongings. Staphysagria easily gets 'pissed off' in a very literal sense.

Insult, mortification and abuse are key concepts to Staphysagria individuals. If an animal falls ill in the months following a new addition to the household, it could be an indication for this remedy. Staphysagria individuals simply don't adapt easily to change.

The remedy's strong affinity with the urogenital sphere, combined with the theme of abuse, puts Staphysagria high on the list of remedies frequently used to treat people who have suffered from sexual abuse. In dogs and cats of both sexes, a couple of doses of Staphysagria is often recommended a few weeks after neutering. I also recommend this remedy on a first aid basis to anyone who has had a urinary catheter inserted, perhaps in connection with treatment for urinary stones.

When cats get stressed, it often translates into physical problems in one of two ways: they react either through the urinary system, with inappropriate urination or even cystitis, or through the skin, often over-grooming to the point of creating bald patches or even wounds (see the chapter on feline cystitis, page 179, and the section on over-grooming, page 164). Staphysagria is often the curative remedy for both types of stress-induced behaviour.

Thuja

Apart from being a constitutional type in itself, Thuja is often used as a specific remedy for warts. Its real claim to fame, however, is undoubtably as the prime remedy against vaccinosis (side effects caused by a vaccine). Having seen time and again how reliably Thuja will cure even life-threatening vaccinosis, I recommend giving this remedy preventatively when anyone (human or animal) is vaccinated (see page 49).

The Thuja type is generally a chilly individual who enjoys a warm environment. They can be quite boisterous and energetic, but more commonly, in my experience, they are quite passive, quiet types. The remedy has particularly strong affinities to the urinary system and skin, especially skin growths ranging from warts and lipomas to malignant tumours.

Sulphur

Sulphur individuals are invariably hot, and will always choose to settle down in the coolest spot available. They tend to be both hungry and thirsty by nature.

The typical Sulphur animal is an easy-going individual who isn't afraid of a bit of dirt; indeed, many seem to positively wallow in it, probably appreciating the cooling properties of mud. They are as far from being sensitive or fastidious as you can get. They may be laid back to the point of laziness or enthusiastically happy-go-lucky in their approach to the world. In either case, they are not a type who worry about themselves or their surroundings.

Sulphur is a very commonly used remedy that, probably more than any other, is prescribed on many different levels. Like Nux vom, it is often employed as a detox remedy, especially after conventional drug treatment, or in cases of parasitic skin problems caused by fleas or scabies (sarcoptic mange).

Sulphur has strong affinities with the digestive system and the skin. It can be helpful on an acute level for treatment of many cases of diarrhoea, and for acute skin infections such as hot spots (see page 162).

Arnica

Arnica has to be the best-known homeopathic remedy of all, and belongs in every home and in every first-aid kit.

Arnica is primarily prescribed as a remedy for physical trauma, with bruising being the main Arnica symptom. There are countless situations where Arnica is invaluable for both people and animals. Give it before and after any surgical procedure, including dental procedures. Any injury, from the slightest knock or sprain to complicated fractures, will heal so much better with Arnica.

Rhus toxicodendron

Rhus tox is a commonly used remedy that is applied at very different levels. As a constitutional remedy, it fits active and energetic individuals. It often suits the headstrong, busy little terrier type, and can, when the type fits, be invaluable in treating the skin allergy he often suffers from.

At a more local level of treatment, Rhus tox has a strong affinity to muscle tissue. Stiffness on first movement is a keynote symptom of Rhus tox in this context. The stiffness improves once the patient limbers up. Whether the muscle soreness and stiffness are due to simple strain and overwork, or more serious and chronic musculoskeletal problems like arthritis, Rhus tox can provide invaluable pain relief, provided this characteristic feature is present.

Often the dog is noticeably lame when he takes the first few steps after getting up in the morning or on the way to the park, but moves more freely once the body has warmed up. After a rest, the stiffness will return.

Although movement helps these patients, it is a fine balance, as over-exertion invariably makes matters worse. Getting up from a few hours of rest after a walk that was really too long is the worst time of all.

One of my homeopathy teachers used to say that everyone who gardens needs a dose of Rhus tox after the first nice spring weekend of the year, in order to be able to get out of bed on Monday morning. Another apt image for the characteristic Rhus tox stiffness is a rusty, creaking gate that moves better once loosened.

With careful observation, it is generally not hard to see the typical Rhus tox aggravations that, apart from rest and over-exertion, are also caused by damp and cold.

Ruta

Ruta's symptom picture is very similar to that of Rhus tox: they share the same aggravating factors. Patients benefiting from treatment with Ruta, like those helped by Rhus tox, will feel a worsening in their symptoms after rest, after over-exertion, and in cold and damp conditions.

Ruta's main tissue affinities are to connective tissue, tendons, ligaments, joint capsules, bone surface, and cartilage. Any patient with an injury to ligaments or tendons should be treated with homeopathic Ruta. Tears, ruptures or weakness of the cruciate

The one homeopathic remedy everyone should know

Arnica is for injury. Any situation in which there is traumatic tissue damage, be it minor or life-threatening, will benefit from this homeopathic remedy. In these situations, picking the correct remedy is easy. If your dog or cat (or, indeed, you) is injured, reach for Arnica. Knocks, falls, bruises, sprains, fractures, traffic accidents, dental procedures and surgery – before you do anything else, give the patient Arnica. You cannot overdose on Arnica in a case of acute physical trauma, so just keep repeating as needed. In a case of elective surgery, such as a spay, I recommend giving a single dose of Arnica 30C the night before, and repeating a single dose the next morning before going to the clinic. Some vets routinely administer Arnica to all surgical patients during procedures, but if yours does not, don't worry about it. Give the two doses before the surgical procedure as described, and resume giving Arnica as soon as you pick up your dog or cat. For the first few days, give at least four daily doses, reducing gradually to one or two daily doses until recovery is complete, typically after about two weeks. Also see page 199 on support around surgery.

ligament of the knee are prime examples of this.

Many cases of musculoskeletal problems, whether acute trauma or chronic cases of dysplasia and osteoarthritis, will have some degree of damage to cartilage or joint capsules, and Ruta will be indicated.

RRA (Ruta + Rhus tox + Arnica)

Homeopathic remedies are generally best given individually. However, the three remedies just described – Arnica, Rhus tox and Ruta – are a rare exception to this rule. They complement one another beautifully, and all are indicated when there is trauma to the musculoskeletal system.

Whether in cases of acute sprain or in chronic osteoarthritis, if the picture as described above fits, combining all three is sometimes the ideal approach.

CASES FROM MY HOMEOPATHIC PRACTICE

Rita

A black, domestic, long-haired kitten born in May 2017, Rita was adopted from a shelter in September 2017 when she was an estimated four to five months old.

Rita came with a tube of antibiotic cream, as the shelter vet, on dismissing her, had noticed a scratch on her nose. Ten days later, the scratch showed no sign of healing, and had, in fact, turned into a sore, with similar crusty sores developing on the edges of both of Rita's ears.

Worried, her new carers took Rita to the local vet, who took a biopsy of one of the lesions. The laboratory biopsy report confirmed that Rita, despite her young age, suffered from a severe autoimmune disorder known as pemphigus foliaceus.

At this point, both the local vet and the shelter vet recommended that Rita be put to sleep as her long-term prognosis was poor, and serious side effects were to be expected from giving the necessary on-going high dose steroid treatment to someone so young. She was put on steroid and antibiotic treatment while the carers considered their options.

Luckily, even though Rita had only been with her new family for a few weeks, the carers had grown very fond of her, and were struck by the fact that she didn't seem ill or in any way affected by the rapidly spreading lesions. They decided to try homeopathy.

When I first met Rita in early November, she had thick, crusty lesions on both her ears and on her nose, but was otherwise bright. She had been receiving high-dose

steroid treatment for a couple of weeks. This treatment was tolerated well but the lesions were still present.

We talked for about an hour while Rita explored my consulting room. In her case this meant bouncing around, throwing herself on the floor, examining every corner, and exploring every surface she could get onto. Greeting both her own people and me briefly in passing, she spent the entire hour actively exploring.

Described as sweet, brave, curious, confident – almost too confident, in fact – and very active, Rita had settled into her new home immediately, and had, according to her carers, been so relaxed that they initially

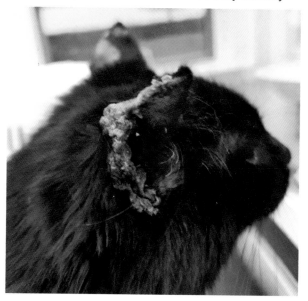

Rita before homeopathic treatment ...

suspected she might be deaf, because even the loudest noise didn't make her jump. She had purred in the cat carrier all the way home from the shelter. Their feeling was that she was surprisingly unafraid. They had been trying to teach her not to scratch the sofa, and described how she completely ignored being told off.

Rita is far from shy. She loves activity, games and company, and is very friendly with

131

guests who come to the apartment. She is affectionate and likes to be held. Rita doesn't appear to feel the cold. She sleeps in bed with her people, but, although she likes close contact, always stays on top of the covers. In the living room, she ignores the cat igloo they bought for her, preferring instead to lie on a cool windowsill.

Based on my impression of Rita, I prescribed the homeopathic remedy Medorrhinum 200C, chosen because it fits Rita's type (constitution) based on, among other things, the above information.

Rita's sores healed within a week of starting this remedy and have never recurred. Rita has needed no further treatment, including steroids, for over a year now, and I think you'll agree she has grown into a beautiful, young adult cat, although sitting still for the camera (or anything else) is still not her thing.

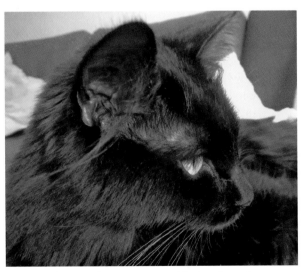

... and after homeopathic treatment.

Toots

Toots is a domestic, short-haired male tabby cat who was born in 2004.

Toots suffered from asthma as well as allergic skin problems that led to over-grooming – in places, to the point of baldness. The asthmatic cough started when Toots was one year old and was, despite long periods of steroid treatment, heard most days for more than ten years. His skin problems started at the age of eight.

Initially, a course of steroids completely stopped the cough, though it invariably returned when the steroid treatment was withdrawn. To reduce the risk of side effects from long-term steroid use, Toots ended up receiving steroids every other day, which reduced the cough somewhat but didn't stop it completely. During other periods, he would only receive his steroid pill when the cough worsened.

As Toots grew older, he began over-grooming to the point that he developed bald spots on his lower back, abdomen, and the inside of his hind legs.

From a young age, Toots had a strong character. He was always an active, bold and curious cat who doesn't accept anyone messing with him or overstepping his personal boundaries. Both his carers and a few vets have suffered his wrath when Toots has felt they were invading his space. His carers describe him as confident and certainly not afraid to send you an angry look. If he feels pushed, he will lash out. Even as a young kitten, if told 'no' or a finger was wagged a at him, he would go for the finger. Too independent to ever be called a lapcat, when handled correctly, he does enjoy the occasional cuddle from his carers. There is a wildness to him, and he will get upset if things don't go his way. As his carers aptly put it, Toots is a 'live wire.'

Toots has always been quite the fastidious cat, and expects his litter tray to be kept clean. No easy task, perhaps, as he has a voracious appetite and practically inhales his food. After a meal, he prefers a cool place to sleep, avoiding the sun and the heater.

For most of his life Toots has been

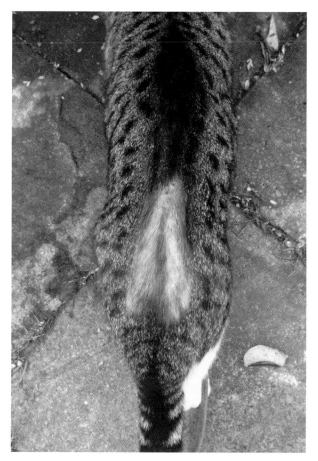

Toots showing severe hair loss from overgrooming.

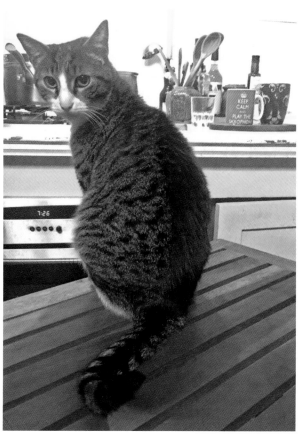

After homeopathic treatment.

treated with homeopathy, herbs and conventional medicine without finding a solution to fully cure his asthma. When his skin issues accelerated, we intensified the efforts, and finally, in the spring of 2015, found the exact match in both remedy and potency when Toots responded beautifully to a single dose of Staphysagria 1M repeated four times at weekly intervals. This remedy was carefully chosen because it fits Toots' personality type and habits. Other cats suffering from allergic skin disease, overgrooming or asthma will need other remedies to find a permanent cure. Finding the perfect remedy for each individual patient is the skill and art of classical homeopathy

Following this treatment, Toots had no more issues with itchy skin, over-grooming or coughing for more than three years. His beautiful glossy coat re-grew, and the cough, which had been heard every day for ten years of his life, resolved. In the summer of 2018, however, his cough began to return gradually, and he started slightly over-grooming the inside of his legs: clear signs that Toots, who had received no treatment of any kind for more than three years, needed a few repeated doses of his curative remedy, Staphysagria 1M.

Toots is now 14 years old and thriving.

Lassie

Lassie is a female Labrador-cross born in 2007.

In July 2016, when she was nine years

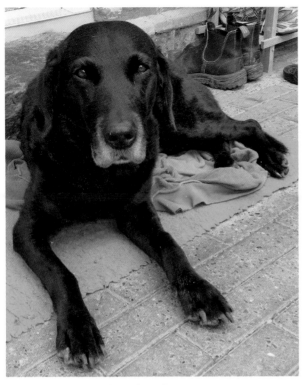

Lassie at home.

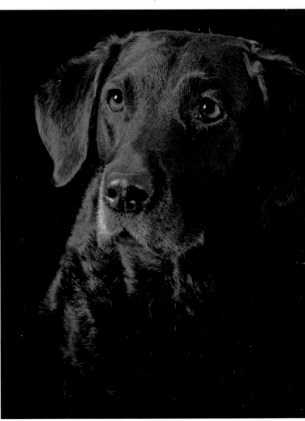

Lassie after homeopathic treatment.

eating and, by Monday, was so bright that the vet couldn't believe it. The planned euthanasia was cancelled.

More than two years later, Lassie is still going strong, and blood tests show no kidney abnormalities. I only met Lassie after her carer saved her life using a simple homeopathy kit. Lassie has received a few different supportive remedies over the subsequent years, primarily to support her pancreas and her joints as she has struggled with geriatric complaints unrelated to the kidney problem that so nearly ended her life.

Lassie remains a happy old lady with a good quality of life.

Fuwa

Fuwa is a female dog of the Japanese Akita breed. Born in 2005 and neutered in 2009,

old, Lassie was dying of acute kidney failure. She was in a collapsed state and on a drip in a referral veterinary hospital. Blood tests confirmed that her kidneys were failing. For those interested in the details, Urea was 32,5 mmol/L (normal reference 2,5-9,6), and creatinine was 310 mmol/L (normal reference 44-159). Lassie did not respond to treatment, so her carers took her home from the hospital on a Saturday afternoon to say a final goodbye, with a plan for a vet to come and put her to sleep on the following Monday morning.

Once home, with no hope and nothing to lose, Lassie's carer, who had no particular knowledge of homeopathy but remembered that she did have a homeopathic first aid kit, consulted the instructions included in the kit, and decided that Lassie's symptoms matched the remedy Arsen alb better than any other. So, she gave Lassie a few doses. To everyone's immense surprise, Lassie quickly and remarkably improved. She got up, started

Fuwa suffered from spay incontinence which began in 2012.

Spay incontinence is a common consequence of neutering in female dogs. It can be treated with conventional medications, but generally also responds well to homeopathy (see pages 80 and 183 about spay incontinence).

At Fuwa's first consultation in 2012, her carer described her as chronically tired or depressed. Even before the onset of urinary incontinence, several vets had been consulted because the committed carer was convinced that Fuwa's lack of appetite and energy must be due to some undiagnosed illness or source of pain, but no other problems had been identified.

Unusually for her breed, Fuwa enjoys cuddling up in front of the fireplace to bask in the heat. She is extremely devoted to her carer but reserved in relation to most other people. If approached, she may bare her teeth and growl in warning.

I prescribed Sepia 200C. This homeopathic remedy suited Fuwa on a constitutional level, as well as being a remedy well-known for its connection to the female hormonal system. Fuwa's energy level and general wellbeing improved immediately.

The dose was later increased to Sepia 1M, given whenever Fuwa's fatigue and low appetite started to return. This happens every few months. Fuwa's urinary incontinence has remained under control for the last six years.

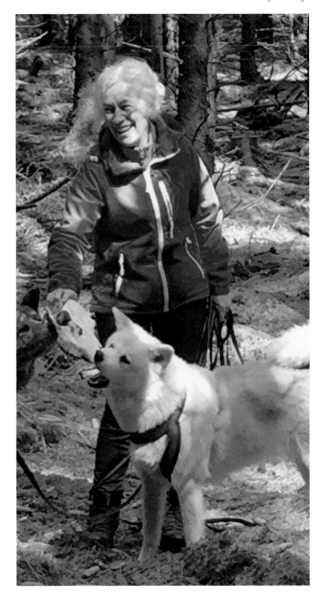

Fuwa exploring with her family.

Fylkir

Fylkir is a male Islandic Sheepdog who was born in 2016. He had no physical complaints but was brought to me to see if homeopathy could help his behavioural challenges. His carers, although highly committed to Fylkir, were struggling (as were their neighbours) with his reactivity and tendency to bark at the slightest provocation.

Fylkir's people had been receiving on-going qualified behavioural help, and had attended training classes since he was a puppy. He had certainly made impressive progress, but, as Fylkir grew up and the constant barking continued, it became clear that something had to change.

Fylkir had a traumatic start in life. His mother and half of his littermates died soon after birth, and Fylkir also came close to death. He, together with three stronger puppies, managed to pull through, and make a full physical recovery.

Fylkir barked at cars. He barked at people. He barked at the TV. He barked if he was left alone and he barked when leaving the house. The slightest sound set him off. If someone popped open a plastic bottle in the kitchen, it would trigger loud barking. His carers described how, once he started barking, it was as if he didn't know that he was doing it, and didn't know how to stop. At home, his restless pacing and panting made quiet evenings impossible.

Fylkir is a sensitive and highly-strung dog. He likes people and is keen to greet everyone, even complete strangers, and if someone is sad, he will comfort them. Fylkir never growls. His carers describe him as sensitive and stressed but never aggressive. Perhaps not unusually for his breed, he doesn't tolerate heat well.

When Fylkir came to see me for the first time in July 2018, I could hear his loud, piercing barking outside the clinic before the car door was even opened. He barked all the way into the building; he barked in the waiting room, and he barked throughout the consultation. He didn't seem scared or threatening in any way. Restless and panting, he walked back and forth between me and his carers to be stroked and cuddled – barking all the while. In fact, after half-an-hour, he was taken outside to make conversation possible.

Homeopaths must, at least briefly, consider the remedy Lachesis for a patient who is quite so loquacious, and who suffers from heat. However, Fylkir doesn't fit the full remedy picture of Lachesis. Instead, I prescribed Argentum nitricum 200C as a good match for his restless, driven, impatient, unable to settle, sociable, open and empathetic personality, together with a few other characteristics.

Within a few days, I received a grateful email saying that Fylkir was transformed.

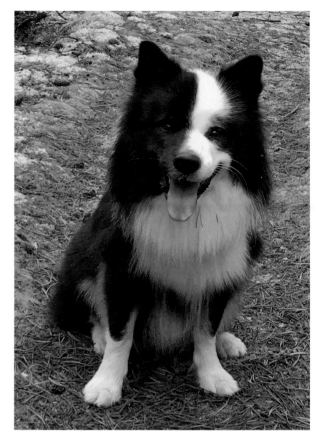

A happy and relaxed Fylkir.

The following month, I opened the waiting room door and was pleased to see a completely silent Fylkir waiting patiently with his carers. After a friendly greeting, Fylkir lay down on the floor of the consulting room for most of the follow-up consultation.

This was very nice confirmation of how homeopathy can supplement the great work achieved through training, as well as give a well-earned break to Fylkir's unusually-committed carers – and their neighbours.

Luna

Luna is a female Alsatian, born in 2011, who suffered from the autoimmune disease lupus.

Luna's symptoms began with lameness in the summer of 2015. She was referred to an orthopaedic specialist clinic where she was scanned and had her joint fluid analysed. She was treated with steroids for a few months. These were eventually discontinued without a return to the previous level of pain, although her carer never felt that she recovered her old personality and energy level.

Sadly, two years later, Luna's joint pains returned with a vengeance, and she also developed ulcers on her nose: another symptom of lupus. Luna's carer was determined that she would not let her go back on steroids, and with euthanasia as the only alternative, it was decided to try homeopathy.

I saw Luna in November 2017 for a homeopathic consultation. While I would normally treat a case of lupus with a carefully chosen constitutional remedy – a homeopathic medicine selected on the basis of the patient's temperament, habits and preferences (appetite, thirst, heat/cold and so on) – I decided, after studying Luna's medical history, to approach this case from a different angle.

I was struck by the fact that her joint pains – Luna's first signs of autoimmune disease – had initially begun soon after she first received two vaccinations against leptospirosis in spring 2015. This led me to suspect that vaccination could have been a trigger for her disease. On this basis, I decided to start treatment specifically against vaccinosis. My plan was to follow this up with a constitutional remedy at a later time, if this was needed. I prescribed the homeopathic remedy Thuja 1M to be given daily for 5 days.

Illness caused as a result of vaccination is termed vaccinosis. While it is often impossible to establish a clear causal link in each case, the fact that autoimmune disease can occur as a direct consequence of vaccination is now well established. Vaccinosis can happen after any vaccine, but most serious cases are believed to occur from the use of killed vaccines, such as those against rabies and leptospirosis.

Luna responded immediately to the

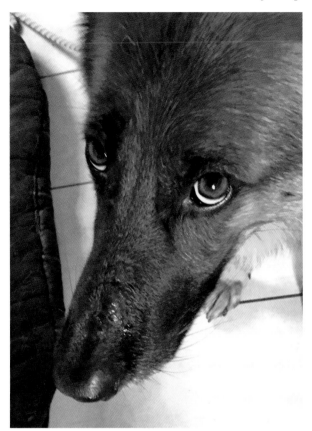

Luna showing ulcers on her nose because of the autoimmune disease Lupus.

homeopathic remedy; two days into the treatment, she was no longer lame. She progressed to make a full recovery over the course of just a few weeks, and she has not been receiving treatment of any kind for nearly two years. There was never a reason to prescribe any other remedy than Thuja.

Her carer is pleased to report that Luna has never been better. Not only are there no physical symptoms of Lupus, a blood test has confirmed that abnormalities could no longer be detected, and the positive changes to her temperament and energy levels are frequently remarked upon.

Luna is clearly a happy, beautiful and healthy dog.

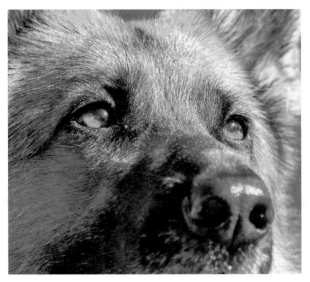

Luna, healthy after homeopathic treatment.

HOMEOPATHY SUMMARY

❖ Take your dog or cat to see a veterinary homeopath if they suffer from allergies in any form
❖ The homeopathic remedy is always prescribed for each individual patient, not just for the condition
❖ Homeopathy can never do harm. It is quite safe to use homeopathy at home

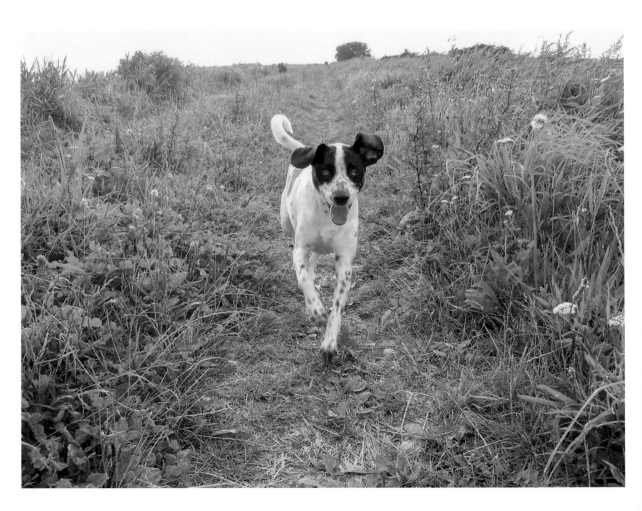

SUMMARY TABLE

	HOMEOPATHY	ACUPUNCTURE	OSTEOPATHY	BACH'S FLOWER REMEDIES	HERBAL MEDICINE
Can I treat my animal?	Yes, but the effect depends on correct remedy	No	No	Yes	Possible with caution
Can the medicine be given with food?	No	n/a	n/a	Yes	Yes
Can it be used in conjunction with conventional medicine?	Yes	Yes	Yes	Yes	Yes
Are there side effects?	No	No	No	No	Yes
For which conditions will it be most effective?	All Treatment of choice for hormonal and immune imbalances (allergies)	All Treatment of choice for locomotor problems (lameness)	Lameness and other locomotor problems	Stress or behavioural problems	All

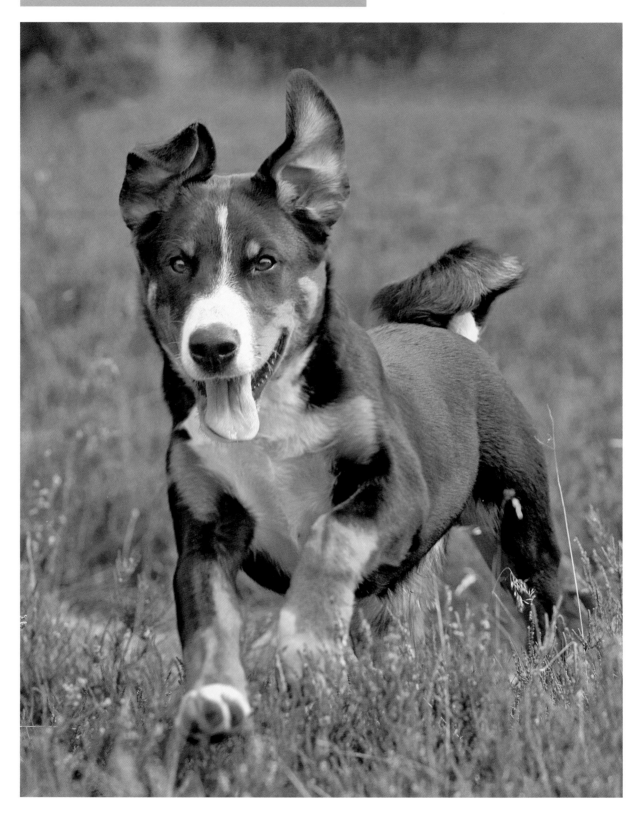

PART THREE
Dealing with disease

Please, please, please, don't lose sight of the main message of this book, which is this: when treating holistically, the treatment is never based simply on the diagnosis. Holistic treatment is always chosen specifically for each and every individual patient.

This means, as discussed in the previous section, that there is no such thing as a homeopathic remedy for a named condition. It means that ten dogs suffering from exactly the same disease will most likely be cured by ten different remedies or treatments. Holistic medicine treats the individual; reductionistic (conventional) medicine treats the disease.

This third and last part of the book discusses specific common health problems, from both a conventional veterinary aspect and a more holistic viewpoint. For ease of use, it is organised in traditional textbook fashion according to organ systems and diagnoses.

This section is most likely to be useful to you if you know an animal suffering from one of the conditions described.

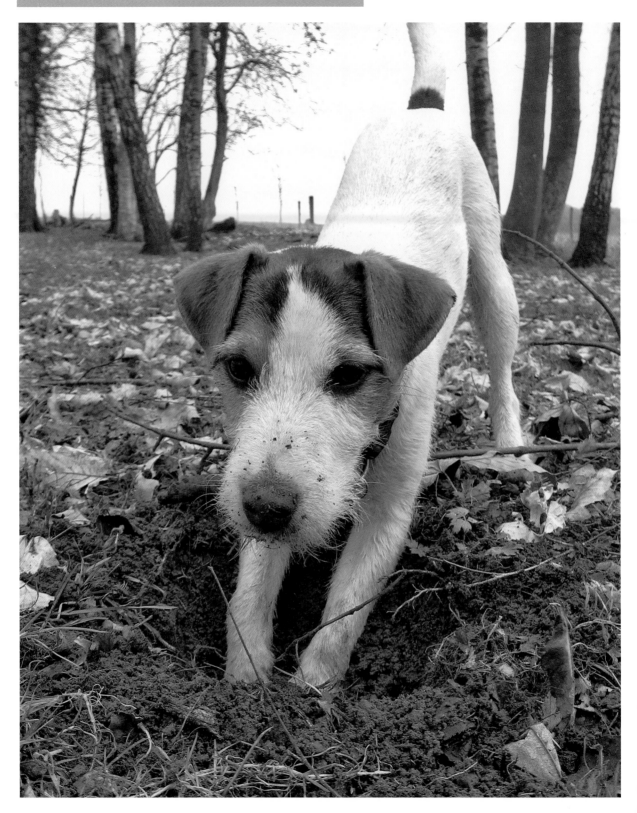

Treat the patient; not the disease

DECISIONS AT THE VET'S: THE RIGHT DECISION IS THE ONE YOU WON'T REGRET

Be aware of all the options

The disease descriptions that make up the rest of this book are in no way an exhaustive list of possible health problems in dogs and cats. I have chosen to discuss a range of common problems because it is my experience that these are conditions where misconceptions are particularly common, or where additional treatments or products can be of such value that both vets and owners deserve to be more aware of them.

I hope to explain the wide range of tools and approaches that are available, and that can often make all the difference, even when dealing with very serious illness.

If your dog or cat suffers from one of the conditions described, I hope the following will help you to feel fully informed when discussing treatment options with your veterinarian, and inspire you to seek further help when relevant.

Each case is different

In many cases, it is possible to argue sensibly for more than one course of action. Make sure, as discussed in the first section of this book (page 37), that you have a vet who is willing and able to listen to you, and who

you trust to be 'on your side' in the decision-making process. There are certainly situations where there is only one responsible way to proceed, but more often there will be different options, and not necessarily one single correct approach. It is even possible to think of situations where one vet would recommend conservative treatment (medication), another surgery, and a third euthanasia.

Your veterinarian has the medical expertise and experience, as well as insight into the specifics of your particular case, and should always be your first port of call. If you hear advice from friends or on social media based on others' experiences in cases that sound similar, ask your vet whether the tips are relevant in your case. Don't try to self-diagnose or self-treat. It is more common than one would think to rely on Dr Google or social media alone, and the consequences can be disastrous.

The elusive truth

Our knowledge is constantly evolving. New diseases are discovered; new treatments introduced. Some areas are still poorly understood, and even for well-described conditions, vets may disagree on the best treatment. 'What we think we know' is certainly not a constant.

The following describes my understanding and my recommendations at the present time. Always listen to your vet: she can no doubt back up her advice. There may be specific factors affecting your case, or new methods may have been introduced. One thing, however, will never change: there will always be decisions that depend on individual values and beliefs about quality of life and the willingness to take risks. Get all your information from reliable veterinary sources, and then make sure that the decisions are your own.

Time to reflect

Good decisions are never rushed, and there are actually very few situations when you must make a decision right then and there, in the consulting room. When possible (and it *is* generally possible, even if this may not be the impression you are given), give yourself some time. I highly recommend that you write down the questions you have, read them out when you are with the vet, note down her answers, and then thank her and tell her that you will go home, consider the information, and return with an answer the next day. Decisions about chemotherapy, surgery, euthanasia, scans, and so on, are only very rarely so time-sensitive that you cannot go home and sleep on them.

It is only natural that your vet may expect the consultation to have a conclusion, and end in a plan of action. Don't get caught up in this. Take away the pressure and remove yourself from the sense of panic and urgency. Simply ask whether the situation will be radically different tomorrow, explain that you would like to sleep on it, and insist on an explanation of exactly how this extra half- or whole day delay is going to affect the outcome. If the surgeon is only available that day, I am sure another clinic will be available next week when you are better prepared. It is not your job to fit into their schedule. You have an important choice

to make, and your responsibility is getting it right for the dog or cat in your care, and for yourself.

The most common situations in which imminent action is needed include a bitch with an acute womb infection (pyometra) requiring immediate treatment, and a male cat who is straining unsuccessfully to pass urine (blocked urethra). In most other cases, even with serious diseases such as cancer, you can afford to take a week to think, talk, sleep, ask questions, and make lists without affecting the final outcome. You may even want to come back for another consultation, bringing along a new list of questions. You may choose to come back with a friend to help you take in the information, ensure that all your questions are asked, and that you understand the answers.

Some vets may feel (and make you feel) that 'now you have all the information, and there is nothing more I can tell you, let us proceed without delay.' I suggest that you take the few extra hours or days to make sure that this is indeed your decision.

FIREFIGHTING

Symptomatic treatment provides short-term relief of symptoms without addressing the underlying problem. I call this type of treatment 'firefighting.' Symptomatic treatment is discussed further in the section on holism (page 101).

Common examples of firefighting include administering steroids or other immuno-suppressive drugs to an allergic animal suffering from a hotspot (acute wet eczema) or an ear infection. In the short term, firefighting certainly has a role to play. An infected ear or hotspot causes intense distress and discomfort, and the treatment brings quick and easy relief that settles things here and now when they are out of control. If the patient has a tendency to suffer recurring ear infections or hotspots, however, and you

Making that difficult decision

- *Write down a list of questions beforehand, and take it with you to the vet*

- *Ask specifically about the expected outcome of all suggested procedures. What is the worst and best that could happen if we do it and if we don't? Write down the answers*

- *Ask how many similar cases they have treated. What were the outcomes?*

- *One more day will rarely make any difference to the outcome. If possible, go home to think about it overnight. Not having to decide then and there removes a lot of pressure*

- *Consider whether it is important to you to pursue all diagnostic tests and know that you have left no stone unturned, or whether you are keen to spare your animal unnecessary discomfort*

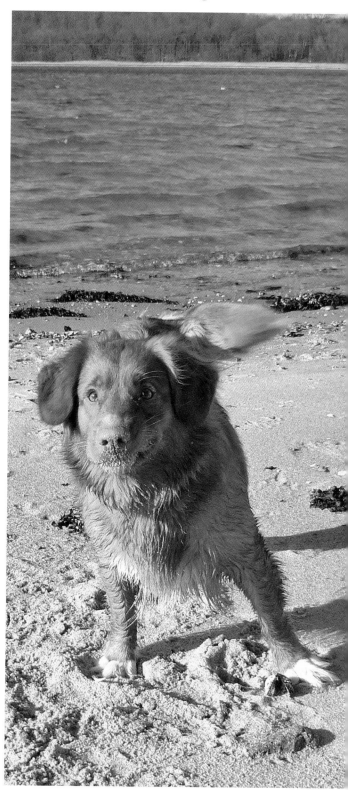

never move beyond symptomatic treatment (firefighting), the problem will keep flaring up: in this example because the underlying allergic problem is never addressed.

Use it, but don't rely on it
I have two things to say about firefighting.

First, don't hesitate to use it when necessary. If there is a fire, put it out. No matter how keen you may be for a deep-acting holistic solution, symptomatic relief is absolutely the right approach if your dog or cat is suffering from an acute problem right now. It is always okay, when you are in the middle of an acute flare-up, to give your animal some short-term relief. It only becomes a problem, if you don't follow up with a more constructive solution, but just keep repeating the symptomatic treatment because the symptoms recur when you stop.

Second, understand that if the same problem keeps recurring, it makes no sense to rely on symptomatic treatments that must be repeated over and over again, or even be given continuously. If your vet believes that there is no alternative to ongoing symptomatic treatment, look up the condition in the following list. There may be other options available (see page 99 about the right tool for the job).

To repeat: firefighting is always okay when needed, but if you don't move beyond this your dog or cat may continue to suffer from the same problem, and never find a cure.

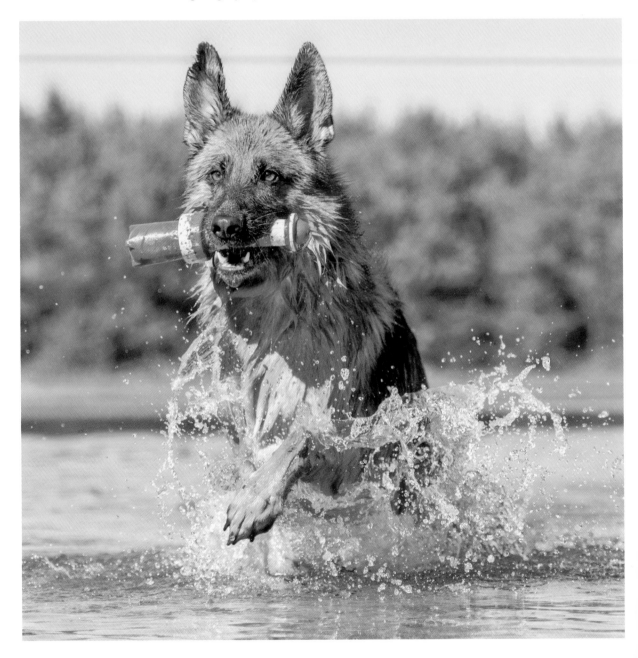

Common conditions in dogs and cats

- Focus on allergy

- Skin
  (Wounds, cat abscesses, eczema, hotspots, ear infections, eosinophilic granuloma complex, psychogenic over-grooming, lumps and bumps)

- Digestive system
  (Dental procedures, gingivitis, vomiting, diarrhoea, constipation, anal sacs)

- Heart and airways
  (Kennel cough, cat flu, asthma, heart disease)

- Thyroid disease
  (Hypothyroidism, hyperthyroidism)

- Urinary system
  (Cystitis, urinary crystals and stones, incontinence, kidney disease)

- Reproductive system
  (Pyometra, cryptorchidism)

- Nervous system
  (Epilepsy)

- Locomotor system
  (Strains and sprains, fracture, cruciate-ligament rupture, dysplasia, osteoarthritis)

- Surgery
  (Aiding recovery)

- Behavioural problems
  (Aggression, fear, car sickness, stress, over-grooming, inappropriate urination)

A problem with a solution

Allergy is a condition in which the immune system is out of balance, and reacts to substances that are not in themselves harmful, so therefore don't cause a reaction in others.

The substances that provoke an immune system in this way are called allergens. An individual can develop an allergy to any substance: a fact that creates a lot of confusion and makes it difficult to compare experiences, as different allergic individuals will react to different allergens. The only thing that all allergic individuals have in common is that their immune system is confused and out of balance, and therefore overreacts to otherwise harmless substances.

Examples of common allergens are grass or tree pollen, house dust or storage mites, and – perhaps less commonly in animals than in people – certain foods. Dogs and cats with unbalanced immune systems tend to overreact to several substances rather than only one or two.

Allergy causes different problems depending on where in the body the allergic reaction happens. A reaction in the eyes and nose causes hay fever, while in the lower airways it causes asthma. In the bowel you get allergic gastroenteritis (IBD), while in the skin you get allergic eczema, resulting in redness and itching.

Allergy is one of the most common health problems in humans as well as in dogs and cats. In animals, unfortunately, allergy tends to take a much more devastating course than it does in the person suffering from hay fever or allergic eczema. One reason for this is that the over-the-counter drugs (antihistamines) that bring relief to many human allergy sufferers rarely have any effect in animals. Allergies in dogs and cats are therefore readily treated with very potent drugs that have serious health implications

On guard!

The immune system is like a soldier standing guard at the entrance to a castle, ensuring that nothing harmful is allowed to enter. The well-functioning immune system holds this post valiantly, and is able to discriminate between what is allowed to enter and what poses a risk and must be stopped. In an allergic individual, the soldier is confused or mad, unable to differentiate between friend and foe, and therefore overreacting, lashing out wildly in all directions, in the process hurting himself and the castle he is supposed to protect.

when used long term. This is why the allergic dog, who is perhaps prone to ear infections or hotspots, ends up suffering much more than you might expect, considering that allergy in itself is rarely life-threatening.

In dogs, allergic gastro-enteritis and allergic skin disease are the most common forms of allergy. Cats also get both of these conditions, and in addition they tend to develop asthma. These conditions are covered in the sections on asthma (page 176), allergic skin disease (page 154), hotspots (page 162), and gastro-enteritis (page 169).

Is allergy inherited?

Nobody knows exactly why someone develops an allergy. Many different factors can damage the immune system; some of them (such as vaccination) are known, while others we don't understand at all. This is true for people as well as for animals. We do know that individuals whose parents suffer from allergies have a higher risk of developing an allergy themselves, meaning that it is certainly possible to inherit a weak immune system.

This is why allergy is particularly common in some dog breeds, although it is not

Allergy alert

An allergy occurs when an individual's immune system mistakenly regards something harmless as a threat. The allergic reaction happens in one or more of the places where the body meets the environment that it is overreacting to –
- *Eyes, nose and throat, causing sneezing and redness*
- *Lower airways, causing asthma*
- *Skin, causing eczema (itchy skin, ear infections, hotspots, paw-licking etc)*
- *Bowel, causing chronic diarrhoea (inflammatory bowel disease, also called IBD or IBS)*

clear cut. You cannot predict that an individual puppy (or kitten or human baby) will develop an allergy simply because one or both parents have allergies; only that he does run a higher risk of it happening. It is also entirely possible for an individual to be allergic when no one else in the family has a problem.

Still, it must be considered unethical to breed from a dog or cat that is being treated for allergic conditions. A responsible breeder will want to be informed if your dog or cat has been diagnosed with an allergy, as this will influence how the parents are used for breeding in the future. This information is crucial for the improvement of the genetic health of your breed, so never neglect to inform your breeder.

Conventional allergy treatments

Allergy cannot be cured with conventional medicine: this is true for people as well as for animals. Your doctor or vet will tell you, therefore, that allergy is incurable, and that the symptoms can only be eased through immuno-suppressive medication. This symptomatic relief works very well in the short term (I call it 'firefighting'; see page 144), but these are very potent drugs, and their long-term use is associated with high risk of serious side effects, making it crucial to limit their use. See page 99 for more on the use of symptomatic treatment as opposed to a cure.

Unfortunately, unlike humans, allergic dogs and cats rarely respond to treatment with relatively mild drugs such as antihistamines. Consequently, potent medicines such as steroids, cyclosporine, and other immune-modulating drugs are needed to relieve the symptoms of allergic disease. Some animals respond to immunotherapy (hyposensitisation), which, in these cases, can help reduce the medication needed. Immunotherapy involves giving the animal increasing doses of the antigens they are reacting to, in an attempt to get their immune system to tolerate them better. In the many cases in which it makes no noticeable difference, the treatment is discontinued in the first year, but for those who show an improvement it is continued for life. Immunotherapy is currently the only conventional approach that aims to treat the underlying allergy. All other treatments are aimed solely at easing symptoms.

Holistic allergy treatments

If I were to choose one area above all others where holistic treatments excel, it would be in the treatment of diseases of the immune system.

As described above, the toolbox available to the conventional vet will not be able to cure an allergic patient. It holds only drugs to keep the symptoms at bay through ongoing suppression of the immune system. This is often tolerated well in the short term but is rarely a safe long-term approach. The fact that many – vets and dog owners alike – are unaware that allergy is curable is one of my chief motivations for writing this book. I am repeatedly frustrated and saddened by hearing of animals being put to sleep because

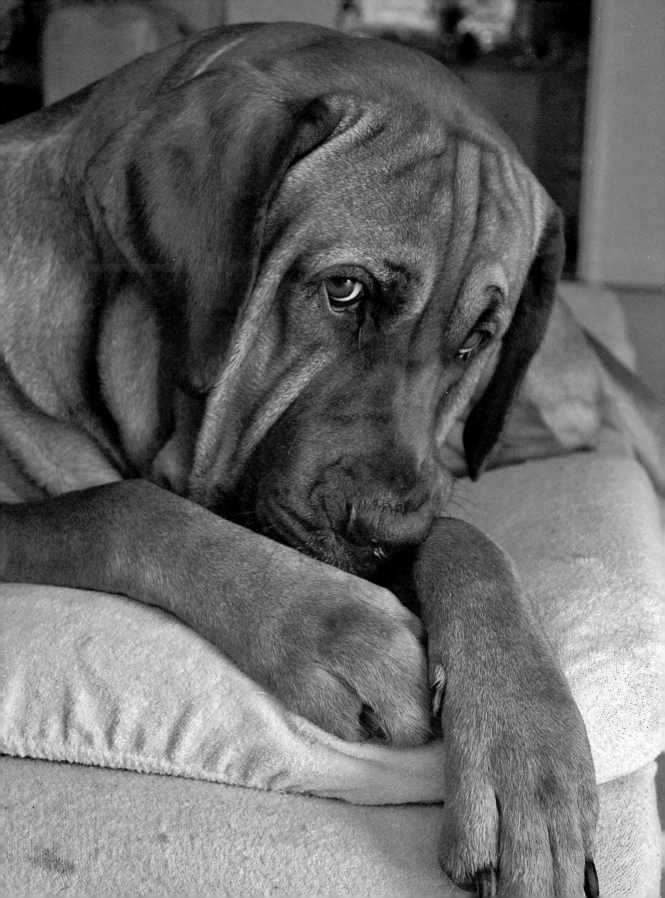

Managing symptoms

An allergic patient receiving ongoing medication to stay comfortable and keep their symptoms at bay has not been cured. The symptoms have merely been suppressed, and it is very likely that the long-term cost to his health will be high.

they suffered from allergies, or by seeing them when they are first brought to me for homeopathic treatment, dying from drug side effects.

Seeing their animals cured after years of ineffective drug treatment, incredulous owners often ask me why no one had told them there were other treatment options? Let me tell you now: holistic treatments, unlike conventional medicine, can, in many cases, cure allergy completely.

If your animal requires treatment for allergic disease, whether it shows itself in the skin, airways or gut, do contact a holistic practitioner. I cannot say it any more clearly. My personal experience is with classical homeopathic treatment of chronic allergy, but an acupuncturist trained in traditional Chinese medicine will also be able to re-balance the immune system. In most cases, this will remove the need for what would otherwise have been a life with ongoing drug treatment.

SKIN

WOUNDS

Wounds may result from various causes, such as bites, scratches, hotspots, over-grooming and furuncles (boils). The general advice given here will be useful in most situations, regardless of the nature of the wound.

Wound cleansing

Cleaning a wound or a scratch on your dog or cat's skin can be done as you would for any other member of the family, with the important difference that you will need to cut the fur. If your patient is not cooperating and you worry about cutting the skin, let your vet shave and clean the area to begin with.

Creams

There are lots of soothing and healing products available. Chances are, you'll have a favourite product: a cream or gel that always works for you as a first aid when you have a rash or a scratch. The temptation to use it on your animals too is easy to understand.

There are plenty of available products aimed at animals, but, as a rule, I don't like them. If you are using an antibiotic or steroid cream to treat an area of skin, naturally, you should continue, and the area will no doubt have been shaved. Otherwise, because animals have fur, any cream, salve or gel is likely to do one of two things.

Firstly, all cats and many dogs will feel that something is sticking to them and attempt to lick it off. Creams are not to be ingested, and licking the area will just worsen the inflammation that the cream was supposed to soothe.

Secondly, because of the fur, most products put on the skin of your animal will stick to the coat rather than being absorbed, which can easily result in matted areas that provide the perfect warm, humid environment in which infections fester and rashes spread.

Soothing or healing creams, great as they may be in themselves, tend not to work on dogs and cats.

Healing with herbs

For the reasons just described, I prefer to avoid non-medicinal creams, relying instead on clipping, cleaning, and preventing the patient from worrying the area, using a collar if necessary.

A great way to cleanse a wound or

scratch is by using the herb Calendula, either as a tea or as a watery dilution of tincture. (Always dilute the tincture, as the neat product will sting.) Add drops of the tincture to a cup of cooled boiled water until a change of colour just becomes visible. Use this solution to rinse the inflamed area. You can bathe the area with the solution, or simply hold a wad of soaked cotton wool against it. Often, the animal will enjoy this.

BITE WOUNDS AND ABSCESSES

Abscesses don't tend to be a big problem in dogs. It happens that anal sacs become infected and form abscesses or that an abscess results from a foreign body, often a grass seed. Cats, on the other hand, excel at producing abscesses.

A catfight will almost invariably result in bite wounds, and bite wounds from a cat almost always turn into abscesses. The entrance wound can be hard to spot, as

the hole left by a tooth is very small and closes easily. It can, however, be deep, and it is always full of bacteria. If your cat (or a neighbourhood cat who crosses his path) is of a territorial disposition, I am sure that you are only too familiar with this problem.

After the battle

Your vet will examine your cat thoroughly after a fight to determine the extent of the damage. If there are signs or a suspicion of bite wounds, she may prescribe antibiotics.

You can follow up this treatment with homeopathic support, and by keeping an eye on any wounds, and, if your cat allows, cleaning them. You can clean a wound using water or whatever product your vet advises, or that you would use on yourself. I like to use a herbal tincture of Calendula (or Calendula mixed with Hypericum) diluted in water as described above in the section on wound cleansing.

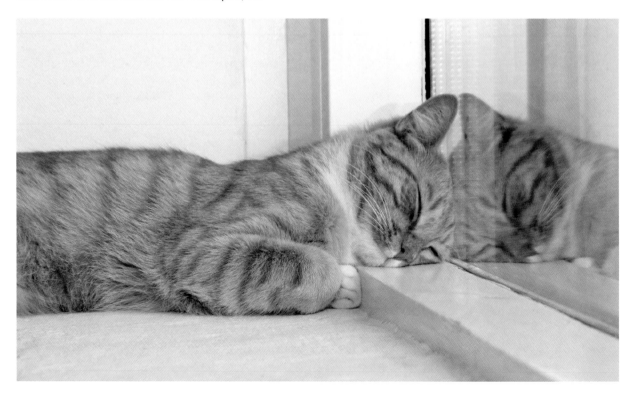

Homeopathic first aid treatment of wounds and abscesses

ARNICA

Always give homeopathic Arnica in any situation involving a physical trauma. Arnica promotes healing and soothes pain in any type of trauma, from the smallest bruise to situations of life-threatening injury or surgery. If a wound occurs from a fight or accident, Arnica is the first remedy to give, as there will invariably be bruising, too.

Arnica is not indicated in the absence of traumatic injury: this means that it is not the right remedy for hot spots or wounds caused by over-grooming, allergic eczema and the like. Arnica is for physical injury only. If your animal has been hit by a car, has had surgery of any kind, has fallen down or has been in a fight, give Arnica 30C several times daily for several days. See page 200

CALENDULA

Just as Calendula in the form of a herbal tincture is excellent for cleaning wounds, homeopathic Calendula will aid wound-healing when given internally. Especially for surgical wounds, large wounds or painful wounds, give Calendula 30C twice daily until the problem is resolved

LEDUM

Ledum is specifically useful for puncture wounds. It can be given before, after, or instead of Arnica for this type of wound

HEPAR SULPH

Hepar sulph is a specific first aid remedy for painful abscesses. Like Arnica and Ledum, this remedy can greatly benefit a cat brawler (and his victims). If the fight has literally just happened, you may be able to prevent infection altogether by giving Hepar sulph in a very high potency (10M). It is more commonly used in a lower potency to help along the process without complications. If you see the fight, or if your cat comes home all ruffled and upset, first give a day or two of Arnica (or Ledum), and follow with Hepar sulph 6C three times daily for a few weeks while any abscesses mature and drain: continue until all is clear.

It is always recommended, of course, that your vet check over your cat, and if there are bites on the face or near joints, or if at any point your cat becomes lethargic, off his food or generally unwell, a vet visit is a must

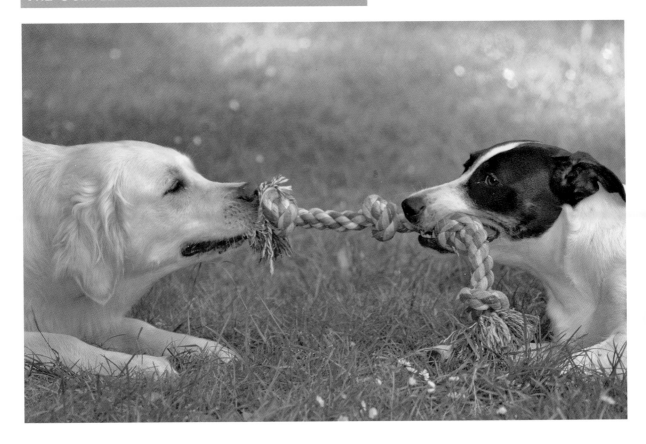

If an abscess is forming, the process can be speeded up by applying a warm compress, as this will help the abscess to mature and open. Several times a day, hold a warm flannel against the area for five minutes or more. If your cat doesn't think this is a great plan, drop it (the plan, that is, not the cat). The area will be painful, and the stress caused by forcing treatment on your cat is both counterproductive and likely to lead to your needing treatment for bite wounds. Some cats are open to this approach, however, so it is worth a careful attempt.

Once the abscess bursts, the problem is solved. You can clean the area if you are allowed; otherwise, just keep an eye on it and on the general wellbeing of your cat. If, at any point, he seems ill, feverish, off his food or in any way not himself, it is off to the vet again.

Never let your cat outside if he is unwell.

Cats tend to hide away – literally to lick their wounds – which means he may be out of reach just when he needs your help. If in doubt, keep him inside, even if he strongly disagrees. It is always better to be safe than sorry.

ALLERGIC SKIN DISEASE

Skin disease caused by allergies is one of the most common conditions seen by any vet in small animal practice. Allergy affecting the skin causes inflammation, and this leads to incessant licking or scratching of the affected area.

Sometimes this reaction is confined to a localised area (often ears or paws), or a well-defined wound (as seen in lick granulomas and hotspots), and in other cases the whole body seems to itch, and the scratching or licking is more generalised. On top of it being one of the most common problems, it is also one of the most frustrating – for the itchy patient, no doubt, but also for the carer as well as for the conventional vet, who, in most cases, will immediately suspect an allergy, and who, of course, is only too aware that allergy is not curable, and so the patient will require ongoing (probably lifelong) treatment. To a vet who knows only conventional medicine, these are true heartsink patients for whom a solution is not in sight.

Atopy

We used to call it 'flea allergy' when dogs or cats licked and scratched themselves raw. Today, we know that the root of the problem is an overreacting immune system, which can cause the patient to react to many different allergens; flea bites being only one of them.

The inborn tendency to overreact in an allergic fashion to allergens in the environment (typically pollen, house dust mites or storage mites) is referred to as atopy, and the sufferers as atopics. Less commonly, animals can develop contact dermatitis or food allergies.

ALLERGY TESTING: WHAT IT CAN AND CAN'T DO

A blood sample (allergy test) is not a way to determine whether someone has an allergy ...
It is a common misunderstanding that a diagnosis of allergy is made on the basis of a so-called allergy test. This is not the case. A vet makes this diagnosis on the basis of a clinical examination, and by ruling out other causes, such as parasites.

There is a blood test available that can check levels of IgE antibodies against common antigens, but, contrary to common belief, this is not done to determine whether the patient suffers from allergies. Firstly, many healthy animals may show elevated levels of IgE in a blood test, making it useless for diagnosing an allergic tendency, and, secondly, no such test

is needed: your vet can make the diagnosis through examining your dog or cat, knowing their history, and ruling out other causes for the symptoms.

... but a way to determine what an allergic patient is reacting to ...
Okay, so although a blood test cannot diagnose someone as having an allergy it has another, very specific use. It is meant to be the first step in a course of treatment known as allergen-specific immunotherapy or hyposensitisation. This is a long-term treatment in which the allergic patient is given repeated minute doses of the allergens they are reacting to in an attempt to lessen this reaction. This approach was common in the treatment of human hay-fever sufferers 40 to 50 years ago.

The blood test (allergy test) is the first step in this course, as it determines how to make up the correct mix of allergens to treat each patient. This is what it can do; nothing else. Still, my impression is that it is often over-used and misinterpreted.

... which is less useful than you might think ...
It would be wonderful if we could establish what an allergic cat or dog overreacts to, and then cure them by removing the offending allergen from their environment. But with the possible exception of pure food allergies, at least for dogs and cats, this doesn't happen. I am sorry, but there it is. If the immune system is out of balance and therefore prone to overreacting, it will overreact to whatever allergens it is exposed to.

In the case of dogs and cats, trees, grasses, flea saliva, mites and moulds are the universal offenders. We can't remove these from the environment to an extent that would make a noticeable difference, and, even if we could, the overreacting immune system would just begin reacting to something else. The problem is with the immune system, not with tree pollen or dust mites.

I know many owners who wear themselves out by incessantly cleaning and washing the house and the dog's bedding. I have yet to see this bring about a significant (or even noticeable) improvement in their animal's allergic symptoms.

Allergen—specific immunotherapy (hyposensitisation)

Some dogs and cats undergoing hyposensitisation experience a notable improvement. Apart from the risk of anaphylactic reactions, this treatment is not associated with side effects, unlike any other conventional allergy treatment. Even though the effect rarely eliminates the need for symptomatic treatment, it is still worth checking whether your dog or cat is among those who can benefit from this treatment, and thus at least reduce the need for other medications. In some cases, immunotherapy combined with fatty-acid supplements and medicinal shampoos can significantly decrease or even obviate the need for more potent medications. Don't continue immunotherapy beyond the first year unless it has had a convincing effect, as will be the case in around half of the animals who start treatment

I had a memorable patient some years ago: a small, itchy dog who, through allergy-testing, had been found to react to house dust mites (as they generally do). The vet had told the elderly woman who lived with the dog that he should no longer be allowed into her bedroom. Following this advice, she moved her bed into the living room, where the dog continued to snuggle up next to her under the covers at night. Although she may have misunderstood the advice, I am convinced that the dog's allergic symptoms were no worse as a result.

Atopy treatment options

- *Essential fatty-acid supplementation*
- *Regular bathing using a medicinal shampoo*
- *Topical cleansing and use of steroid/ antibiotic cream (as needed to stop inflammation or infection without systemic drugs)*
- *Hyposensitisation (ongoing if a positive effect is seen after a trial period)*
- *Systemic short courses of antibiotics and/or steroids during flare-ups*
- *Continual use of potent immune-suppressive drugs such as steroids, oclacitinib (Apoquel) or cyclosporine (Atopica)*

The above list is intended as a 'ladder.' Start at the top at the first sign or suspicion of allergy. As the need for further treatments arises and you move down the list, I strongly recommend consulting a veterinary surgeon with experience in homeopathy or acupuncture. See pages 98 and 215

... except as part of immunotherapy

So, the blood test that is commonly referred to as an allergy test has one use and one use only: as the first step of the treatment known as immunotherapy. For everything else, it is useless. If you are not planning or even considering a course of immunotherapy, it makes no sense to do the test.

Immunotherapy is the only approach within conventional medicine that aims to reduce the sensitivity of the immune system to certain allergens. Unfortunately, it is not always very effective.

The typical approach is as follows. Once you have established that your dog or cat has an allergy that requires treatment, a blood test is done. If this shows raised antibody levels to a certain number of common antigens, a preparation of these is manufactured specifically to suit your animal. This can be given either as injections at increasing intervals or as drops given orally every day on an ongoing basis.

After nine to 12 months of this treatment (without any symptomatic treatments confusing the picture), you sit down with your vet to assess the response. If there has been no improvement or only very limited improvement, the treatment is dropped. If there has been sufficient improvement that warrants ongoing treatment, it is continued for the rest of the animal's life.

From my experience, somewhere around a third to half of patients who start treatment find it beneficial enough to continue. In most of these cases, ongoing immunotherapy alone will not cure all of the symptoms, but it can alleviate them enough to reduce the need for other medications, and thereby reduce their side effects.

In conclusion, this is the safest and most constructive approach to allergy treatment within the realm of conventional medicine. It is, however, not very effective: it can, in roughly every other allergic patient, contribute to a lessening of symptoms. I therefore find it worth doing, but don't be surprised if (after a lot of doses) it turns out to have had little or no effect, and do be aware that holistic medicine can offer treatments that provide much better odds.

If professional holistic therapy is not available, I would certainly advise against ongoing immune-suppressive medications such as steroids, cyclosporine or oclacitinib (Prednisolone, Atopica, Apoquel or other trade names) without having first taken the trouble to determine whether immunotherapy can reduce the need for these potent drugs in your animal. In rough numbers, allergen-specific immunotherapy (hyposensitisation) can halve the discomfort in half the patients.

Diagnosing food allergy

Although finding out what an allergic animal is reacting to sounds like a sensible and constructive approach, it's actually, as already mentioned, surprisingly unhelpful.

Atopic patients react to allergens in the environment, and we can never control these enough to make a significant difference. The one situation in which we can decide what an animal is exposed to, however, is when it comes to food. Even though only a very small minority of allergic dogs are allergic to food, it is certainly worth knowing whether your dog is one of them, as this is the one situation where you can easily take steps to avoid the offending allergens.

Dogs and cats can develop allergies to any food they are exposed to. It takes a while to become sensitised, so the allergy will be to foods that they have eaten without problem for some time, not to something they are being offered for the first time.

The most common food allergens for dogs are beef, chicken, eggs, dairy, wheat, soy and corn. For cats, the top offenders are chicken, fish and dairy. This statistic doesn't

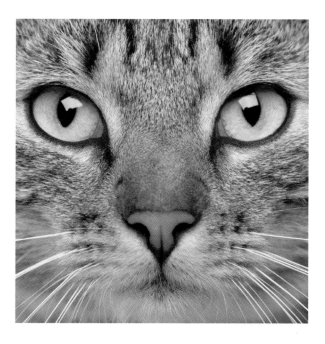

mean, of course, that your allergic dog should not have beef or chicken. You need to establish first, if your dog or cat has a food allergy at all, and, if so, what food item or items he is reacting to.

An elimination diet trial is the only definitive way to diagnose a food allergy. Other tests based on blood or saliva do exist but are controversial. If you have a dog with an allergy, and you would like to know whether the diet you feed can affect it, here is what you do.

Elimination diet trial

To determine if a food allergy could be why your dog or cat suffers from allergic skin disease, you need to carry out a strict diet for three months – and by strict I mean stricter than strict. You learn nothing at all by just feeding less of a certain food, or by assessing day-by-day or week-by-week how your dog is reacting to changes in diet. If you want to know if diet is relevant to your animal's allergic symptoms, and you are going to do the trial, do it properly.

The first step is deciding to do a food trial. It is a hassle, for sure. For a period of three months, you need to ensure total control of every crumb your dog eats or even chews on – but remember that it is not a permanent new diet. It is simply a temporary inconvenience for a specific purpose: namely, to provide very useful information about your dog or cat's allergy.

Once you are committed to doing the trial, the next step is deciding what to feed. You need a simple diet consisting of one or two components that your animal is very unlikely to react to. This can be done in one of two ways. You can provide a so-called novel protein source: in other words, a vegetable protein or type of meat that your dog or cat has never been exposed to before, and therefore cannot have developed an allergy to. The other approach is to feed a processed hydrolysed diet. This is typically in the form of

a dry food where, during the manufacturing process, the ingredients have been broken down into fragments that are too small for the immune system to recognise as allergens.

Some experts recommend fresh novel protein as the optimal approach of the two, as some allergic animals will react even to a hydrolysed diet. I have often carried out food trials using a home-made diet of horse meat and sweet potato, but any meat that your animal has never tasted before can be used, and exotic meats such as rabbit, kangaroo, alligator, ostrich, and even insects can be used as the protein source during the trial. Choose one that your dog or cat will eat, and stick to it for the three months of the trial.

During this trial period, your dog must ingest nothing at all apart from the selected diet food. No toothpaste, no treats, no chews, no exceptions. Also, avoid any supplements and, when possible, medicines during the trial, as flavourings and gelatine capsules may contain soy, pork or beef allergens. Watch out for pitfalls such as scavenging behaviour (some dogs can complete a trial only by wearing a muzzle), friendly dog lovers in the park sharing treats before you have time to shout NO, small children dropping food or kindly grandmothers sharing a secret treat.

Needless to say, it is particularly difficult

to carry out an elimination diet if there are several animals in your home. The easiest solution may be to put them all on the same diet. There is no point in a gradual diet change, as is generally recommended when changing diets. For this purpose, simply switch over from one meal to the next.

A diagnosis of food allergy is made by first demonstrating that your animal's symptoms clear up (without medications) during the trial, and then that they return when you re-introduce the problematic food item. You can, of course, simply put them right back on their old diet to test for a recurrence of symptoms. If the problem returns, you have achieved the point of the trial: namely, to confirm that your animal has a food allergy, and that adjusting the diet is the way to go.

If, at the conclusion of the diet, your dog or cat has seemingly responded well and has no symptoms, however, you could choose to introduce one food item at a time at a rate of no more than one new pure food per week. In this way, you will not only discover that a food allergy is present, but also what foods to avoid. While it takes up to 12 weeks to clear a reaction, it takes only a few hours or days to bring on a reaction if he is fed something he is already allergic to. I suggest introducing, say, chicken with most meals (of the elimination diet food) for seven to ten days. If no reaction occurs, chicken is fine, and you can, week-by-week, proceed to test beef, cheese, and so on.

What then, if you diligently carry out a three-month diet trial, swear on your life that your dog has not eaten a smidgen of anything other than the chosen diet food, and still there has been no improvement in his skin symptoms? Was it all a gigantic waste of time and effort?

Far from it.

This is by far the most common outcome of an elimination diet trial (remember that the vast majority of allergic dogs don't suffer from food allergies), but it is still totally worth

doing it. Provided, of course, that the diet was strictly adhered to, and that your animal wasn't reacting to the diet itself (as can be the case with hydrolysed diets), a lack of response demonstrates that your dog is allergic to environmental allergens, and not to food. This means that you can forever forget about diet in relation to the allergy. No more money wasted on expensive allergy foods. You now know that, in your case, diet doesn't come into it.

What is the best diet for an allergic dog?

I hope that, by now, you appreciate how little sense this question makes. The answer, of course, is that if the dog belongs to the majority of allergic dogs who are allergic to environmental allergens rather than to food, it doesn't matter (in this context) what he eats. He is not allergic to his food. If, on the other hand, he is one of the minority and does have a food allergy, the answer to the question depends entirely on what food the dog in question is allergic to, and the only way to know whether your dog has a food allergy (and, if so, what foods he should avoid) is to carry out an elimination diet trial.

Food for thought

A large majority of allergic dogs and cats are allergic not to food but to allergens in the environment, such as grass, pollen, fleas, moulds, house dust mites, and storage mites

Who you gonna trust?

It is my impression that the subject of diet and its relation to allergies is particularly plagued by confusion and false claims. For the reasons explained above, you should not expect another dog owner's experience to be relevant or helpful. Also, raw meat or grain-free diets cannot with any validity be marketed (as they often are) as 'allergy-friendly.' A raw meat diet may help a dog suffering from a food allergy to wheat or soy, but it won't, of course, help a dog with a food allergy to the meat they are being fed. And, as we know, most allergic dogs aren't allergic to food at all.

Storage mites

It does seem to be the case that more than the few we would expect (because only a small minority of allergic dogs have a food allergy) do experience improvement when taken completely off dry foods. The explanation for this most likely has to do with storage mites, a very common environmental allergen.

Storage mites will be present in all dry foods and chews. I strongly suspect that many dogs get better after a complete switch from dry food, treats and chews to either a home-cooked or a raw diet simply because they are no longer exposed to storage mites. Reaction to storage mites is much more common than food allergies. It is not a food allergy, as it is not a reaction to the food ingredients, but rather to the mites that are present because the products (kibble, chews, and the like) have been dried.

Why is there so much talk of allergy diets?

I think there are several reasons for the disproportionate focus on diet in relation to allergic dogs and cats. I say 'disproportionate' because the vast majority of allergic patients won't have a food allergy at all. Even so, the first thing most vets do when they suspect an allergy is reach for the allergy food that fills every vet's waiting room.

Why?

First of all, allergy is an incredibly frustrating condition (for owner, patient and vet). It is easy to be overwhelmed by a feeling of helplessness, knowing that it will most likely never be resolved. The cost to the patient's long-term health from the potent drugs needed to secure a comfortable life doesn't bear thinking about when you are presented with an itchy puppy. The vet wants to help, but in most cases doesn't have the tools.

Changing the diet is at least *something* we can do. And, as described above, a small proportion of allergic patients will be helped by diet changes, so it is absolutely worthwhile to identify them.

It seems to me, however, that many (animals and owners) are living with imposed diet restrictions and expenses without any sense or reason behind them, because of the invalid reasoning that 'your dog is allergic, so he should eat allergy food.' Starting any kind of hypoallergenic diet is nonsense unless it is done as part of a properly carried out elimination diet trial. Feeding an 'allergy diet' without knowing if your dog has a food allergy, and maybe even while still feeding processed treats and chews or supplementing the diet with scraps, will have no effect. None.

A second reason that this is nonetheless a very common story is, I believe, that on first suspicion of allergic disease, a vet may have prescribed a short course of steroids to break the itch cycle, and reached for a bag of hypoallergenic food. For years to come, the owners, who perhaps never got the long explanation about allergy and diet, or didn't take it all in, remember only that the itch did get better when they started the diet (doubtless due to the accompanying steroids), and without proper discussion or explanation they simply keep buying it for years. An allergic dog needs allergy food ... right?

Veterinary prescription allergy diets

Most veterinary clinics offer a selection of prescription diets to be used as part of the treatment of various illnesses, and allergy diets have got to be among the top sellers.

As described in the section on elimination diet trials, allergy diets contain a limited number of ingredients in order to reduce the risk of allergic reactions. The ingredients are hydrolysed, meaning

Allergy and vaccination

The manufacturer's informational leaflet that accompanies any vaccine always states that only healthy animals should be vaccinated. This should be strictly adhered to. Current vaccination guidelines mean that adult dogs and cats only rarely need to be vaccinated in any case (see the chapter on vaccination, page 42). Even when a vaccine is due, I suggest that you be careful about the timing of it. Remember that an allergic animal has a sick immune system. A vaccination may not even work (especially if immuno-suppressive medicines are being given at the same time), but, more importantly, any vaccine is a strain on the immune system, and may worsen the allergic condition

the constituent food items are turned into fragments so small as to be unrecognisable to the immune system. Allergy diets can be used in elimination diet trials, and, for those who respond (meaning that they do have a food allergy), they can be continued long term.

Nutrition is important, of course, and a high-quality diet is always a good thing, but, for an allergic animal with no food allergy, removing (or, for that matter, adding) specific food items won't make the slightest difference to his allergic symptoms. Avoiding storage mites by cutting out anything dried may help. Even dried allergy diets have a role to play, but they are often used without proper understanding, meaning that many allergic animals are on strict diets for years and years, even though it makes no difference to their symptoms, and comes at great cost to their carers.

Treatment of allergic skin disease
See the beginning of this chapter, where the benefit of holistic treatments for allergic

disease (page 149) and the difference between cure and symptomatic treatment (page 145) are discussed, and the section on firefighting (page 144).

It is worth testing whether a complete switch to a home-cooked or raw diet that avoids all dry food, treats and chews makes a difference. This is not the same as an elimination diet trial. Avoiding dried products will help if a reaction to storage mites is a major part of your animal's allergy, meaning it will help some and make no difference to others.

To determine whether your animal has a food allergy, consider an elimination diet trial as described on (page 158).

Supplementation with fatty acids (omega 3) supports the skin and coat. Plant-based oils such as evening primrose are currently recommended over fish oils when the aim is to benefit the skin and coat. It is important that the oil is of a high quality. Choose a reputable brand, buy a small bottle, and store it in the fridge to ensure freshness. A rancid oil will do more harm than good.

Other plant-based oils, such as olive or rapeseed, will not have the same beneficial effect. Oil is food rather than medicine, so you don't have to worry unduly about dosage. Add a teaspoon to a small dog's food, and up to a tablespoon for a large dog. You can also share the oil with your dog (it is great in salad dressings or smoothies, but not suitable for cooking); that way the bottle will be used up more quickly after opening and you can move on to a fresh supply. Essential fatty acid (EFA) supplementation will not cure an allergy or an itch, but it will help support the skin, and after about a month you should notice an improvement in coat quality and shine.

In summary, determine whether diet changes are relevant. Feed a high-quality, plant-based oil. Use shampoos, creams, antibiotics and immune-suppressive medications (such as steroids) for short term relief (firefighting) when needed, and consult an holistic vet with the aim of finding a long-term cure. If a holistic vet is not available, and ongoing immuno-suppressive medication becomes unavoidable, consider immunotherapy (hyposensitisation) as an attempt to lower the dosage needed to keep symptoms at bay.

HOTSPOTS

Hotspots are painful wounds that appear very suddenly. They are mostly seen in long-haired dogs, and tend to happen during hot and damp weather, but any dog can develop a hotspot at any time.

A hotspot is a moist wound that can appear and grow to a significant size within hours. There may be nothing wrong when you leave in the morning, but, when you return in the afternoon, your dog is cowering in pain, his fur sticking together in a wet, smelly, infected area. Hotspots are sometimes seen after tick bites or scratches in the skin. If a dog suffers from recurring hot spots, it is most likely due to an underlying allergic problem.

Treatment of hotspots
Your vet will shave and clean the affected area, and supply a collar to prevent your dog from licking or scratching the wound. You will be instructed on how to clean the wound at home, and probably given an antibiotic cream.

Antibiotics and steroids, either as an injection or in tablet form, are sometimes given as well. The most important step by far in the treatment of recurring hotspots is to shave or cut all fur from the area. Wet, sticky hair adhering to the skin is the optimal environment for infection. You want air to get in. The wound may be too painful for your dog to allow you near it, or too large to tackle with a pair of household scissors. When in doubt, always see your vet.

Many owners of dogs with recurring hotspots do learn to deal with these at home. Preventing your dog from reaching the area, shaving or cutting off all fur in the area, and cleaning the wound several times a day are the important steps. The wound needs to dry out and be exposed to the air. For this reason, aloe vera or other soothing ointments are not a good idea. Shave it, clean it, and then leave it – and made sure your dog does, too.

If you don't go for antibiotics and steroids in the first instance, keep a very close eye, as these wounds can develop quickly and be very distressing for your dog. Hotspots are acute infections, and generally heal almost as quickly as they appear, provided the area is exposed to the air and left in peace.

If they keep coming back, you need to deal with the underlying tendency, as described in the previous pages about allergic problems.

EAR INFECTIONS

Cats with ear infections probably have ear mites. One visit to the vet and the problem should be solved.

Many dogs, on the other hand, suffer repeated ear infections, and often the underlying cause is an allergy. This means that, even though the problem seems to be isolated to one or both ears, it is likely to be an expression of a deeper immune imbalance (allergy) that needs to be addressed if you hope to ever put the problem behind you.

Treatment of ear infections
Your vet needs to examine the ear canal before and after each course of treatment
Your dog is scratching his ears or shaking his head. Perhaps you can even see that the ear opening is red and inflamed, or that the ear canal is full of black or brown secretions.

Get him to a vet. Trauma to the earflap from all the shaking and scratching can burst the small vessels inside the earflap, and then you have an ear haematoma (blood blister) as well as an ear infection. Even more importantly, neglected ear infections easily lead to chronic changes that can make it very difficult to ever fully restore normal conditions inside the ear canal.

A proper examination is important for several reasons. Your vet needs to check if the eardrum has burst or is still intact, as well as rule out the presence of a foreign body, such as a grass seed or lump of earwax or hair, that may need to be removed.

When the exact cause of the irritation has been established, it is possible to start targeted treatment, which greatly reduces the risk of your dog developing a chronic infection that may become resistant to treatment. For these reasons it is absolutely not recommended that you treat an itchy ear with whatever broad spectrum eardrops you may have lying around from last time rather than having the ear examined and properly treated. In some cases, the ear may be so painful that your dog will need to be sedated

for a full examination and flushing of the ear to be possible.

I think it is easy to underestimate the importance of proper examination and treatment of each case of itchy ear inflammation. There are simple ear infections, of course, where all it takes is the right drops for a week or so (although you should always have the ear checked again at the end of the course to make sure that the condition has cleared up fully, and that it is safe to stop treatment). But, when an ear infection recurs for a second or third time, it is no longer sufficient to just apply the same broad spectrum product. You'll wind up in a vicious circle until the ears are permanently inflamed and the drops no longer work.

Treat the underlying cause

Any dog can get a single episode of ear infection, and there is no need to make a big deal of it (beyond having it examined and effectively treated). If it becomes a recurring problem, however, it needs to be taken more

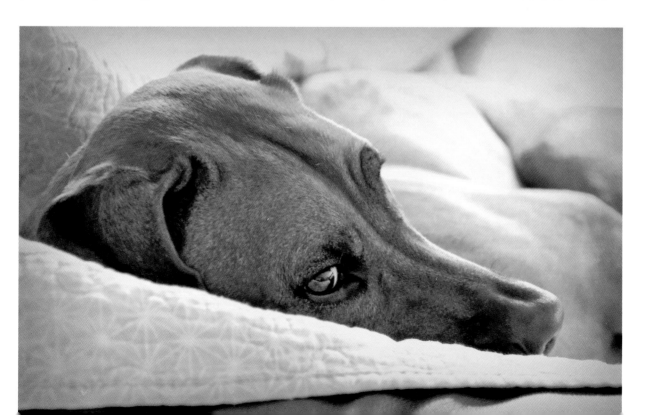

seriously (as I have just described) to avoid chronically inflamed and damaged ear canals.

Some vets will refer to a dermatologist at this point. At the very least, it is important to select the appropriate antibiotic treatment and ensure that the ear is clear before ending treatment. The common approach of many owners of dogs with 'problem ears' – using a broad acting product for a few days until the itch subsides for now – is the straight road to long-term problems.

As important as it is to ensure proper local treatment to preserve the integrity of the ear canal, the most important aspect of dealing with chronic ear problems in dogs is addressing the underlying cause. Hypothyroidism may be the culprit, but another, and the most common, is allergy.

Sometimes an allergy expresses itself as a generalised skin problem, involving the ears as well as other parts of the skin, but, in many cases, ear problems may be the only signs of an allergy. Cure the allergy (see page 101), and the ears will be fine.

EOSINOPHILIC GRANULOMA COMPLEX

A skin disease of cats. The name refers to the type of immune cells (eosinophilic leucocytes) that are found in a biopsy of the lesions that accompany this condition seen only in cats.

The underlying cause is an imbalanced immune system, as with any other allergy, and symptoms vary. Some cats get only a raised ulcer on their lip, by the incisor: a so-called 'rodent ulcer.' In more severe cases, there are one or more raised masses or ulcers on the body and legs. The cat is very bothered by these ulcers, licking them incessantly, whereas a rodent ulcer on the lip often doesn't seem to cause much discomfort.

Treatment of eosinophilic granuloma complex
The conventional approach to this condition is as described for any allergy. A food elimination trial can be carried out to determine whether there is a food allergy. Immune therapy can be started to see if it makes a difference. Most, if not all, of the cats will need long-term immuno-suppressive medications such as steroids to keep symptoms at bay.

As with all other conditions caused by an imbalanced immune system, I highly recommend holistic treatment such as homeopathy or acupuncture. If your cat is already receiving ongoing immuno-suppressive treatment for this condition, don't worry. It is never too late to contact an holistic veterinary surgeon. See the information at the back of the book on how to find a practitioner.

PSYCHOGENIC OVER-GROOMING

Cats are famously clean animals, and their daily healthy grooming ritual involves licking to make sure (one assumes) that every hair is in place. Sometimes this normal behaviour turns into almost manic licking of the same area, to the point where it starts breaking hairs, and possibly even creating bald spots. The abdomen, groin area and legs are most commonly affected.

We talk about psychogenic over-grooming when we have ruled out other causes, such as parasites, infection, generalised itch, pain or neurological disorders. These cats don't have fleas or eczema or any other physical reasons, that we can identify, for the constant licking. They are not, as an allergic cat would, licking in response to a problem with the skin. It is the other way around. They are creating a problem with the skin and coat through licking. Some cats continue this exaggerated licking of the same spot even after all the hair has gone, proceeding to break the skin and create large ulcers.

My feeling is that it isn't always clear whether this is purely a psychological problem or, at least in part, a physical one, but, if you look holistically at the problem, the two are not mutually exclusive. It can be difficult to completely rule out a physical cause, but this is a fairly common condition in cats, many of whom are eventually diagnosed as suffering from a stress-induced obsessive-compulsive disorder.

Treatment of psychogenic over-grooming

It is possible to simply rely on long-term use of psychotropic medications, but I think we can all agree that this should be a last resort, and that all other options, including finding a new home for the unhappy cat, should be considered first.

It is crucial to try to understand why your cat is stressed. Did the behaviour start after changes in your living conditions? Are you stressed? Psychogenic over-grooming can be seen in any type of cat, but it is more common in oriental breeds. Some individuals are just more sensitive than others. Some cats don't thrive without outdoor access. Some cats don't thrive in a household with other cats. Don't blame yourself, but do try to understand your cat. Could the behaviour result from boredom, loneliness, or perhaps overcrowding in a multi-cat household? Is there conflict between cats in the house or in the neighbourhood? Can the living space be improved? Are there enough high perches and hiding places? Are there enough litter trays? Are the litter trays and food bowls too close together? Are they in places that feel safe to the cat? Either your vet or a cat behaviourist can help you to look at your home and make it safer or more stimulating, depending on the specific situation.

Install a pheromone diffuser (see page 214) in the room where the cat spends most of his time. There are also calming food supplements (see page 210) that help many cats, and which, together with changes to the environment or lifestyle of the cat, must be tried before medication is even considered.

As you can see, much can be done

to help a cat who is suffering from stress. Bach flower remedies, homeopathy and acupuncture can often be curative by strengthening your cat, and helping him to overcome his mental or emotional sensitivity.

See more about cats and stress in the chapter on cystitis on page 179.

LUMPS AND BUMPS

Warts, cysts, growths, fatty lumps, cancers – in short, tumours of all sorts – are common in dogs, and cause a fair deal of confusion. When to react, when to worry, and when to calmly ignore and let be?

Any kind of lump is called a tumour, regardless of the type of tissue involved. Tumours can be benign (harmless) or malignant (cancerous). No one – I repeat, no one – has the magical power of being able to look at or feel a tumour and say whether it is benign or malignant. Not even the most experienced vet in the world possesses such insight. The only way to competently assess a tumour is by looking at a sample of it through the lens of a microscope.

Malignant tumours are the same as cancer, whereas benign tumours are completely harmless, unless their size and position mean that they get in the way of normal movement, put pressure on other structures, or in some other physical manner simply get in the way. It is clear, then, that we want to remove malignant tumours as quickly as possible, and that we can safely leave benign tumours unless they are very large or in a problematic area.

The problem is knowing which is which, and a tissue sample from the lump is the way to find out. This can be done either by taking a very small sample (needle biopsy) with a syringe, or by removing a larger section of the lump (or indeed the whole thing) during a small surgical procedure under full anaesthesia.

There are pros and cons to both

approaches: let your vet guide you about the best way to proceed in your case. Removing the complete lump has the prime advantage of making a clear diagnosis easy. The laboratory will have plenty of intact tissue, and should be able to identify the cells of the tumour with no difficulty. Fine-needle biopsies, by their nature, remove only a few cells, which may not be representative of the whole tumour, and which, furthermore, may become damaged in the process, leading to an inconclusive result. Some experts believe that the process of taking a biopsy may have the unfortunate effect of spreading or activating the cancer, should the tumour turn out to be malignant.

If the whole lump is removed in the first instance, the thing is done and, no matter what kind of cells are found, there is no need for further surgery. On the other hand, there are situations in which the surgeon prefers to know beforehand what type of tumour she is dealing with, and therefore may recommend a biopsy before contemplating surgery. It can be helpful to know, especially if operating in an area where healing may prove difficult, whether the tumour is malignant; if so, it is important to make a wide incision to ensure full removal.

Another scenario is that the vet may suspect that the tumour is benign and want to confirm this in order to spare an old or weak patient invasive surgery that may not be necessary.

THE DIGESTIVE SYSTEM

OPEN WIDE

Most dogs and cats will, at some point, need to go in for a veterinary dental procedure. It is not possible to examine the mouth of a dog or cat properly without full anaesthesia, because, unlike humans at the dentist's, even the nicest dog will be disinclined to lie down and open wide for half-an-hour. Typically, you will drop

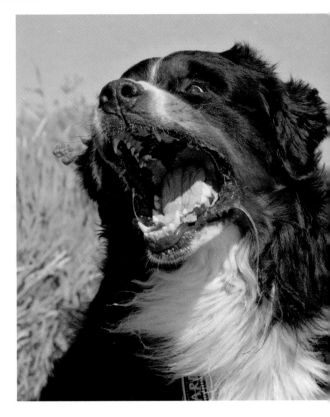

off your animal in the morning, and pick him up again in the afternoon when the anaesthesia is wearing off. The dental procedure may be a routine clean, scale and polish to remove plaque and tartar build-up in order to maintain good oral hygiene, or there may be a suspicion of problems that need to be investigated. Perhaps teeth have even decayed to the point that they need to be extracted.

Undergoing anaesthesia is not to be taken lightly. The risk that most owners ask about and fear – that their animal will not wake up again – is so small for these planned procedures that it shouldn't be a cause for concern. I have no doubt, however, that anaesthesia takes its toll on the body (not least the brain), and should not be repeated needlessly. Rotten teeth and inflamed gums are painful, and can be the root of more serious disease, so if a dental procedure under full anaesthesia is needed, of course it must be done. In many cases, though, these problems can be prevented.

An appropriate diet will go a long way toward ensuring good dental health. See page 33 on the benefits of feeding bones.

It is, of course, possible to brush your dog's or cat's teeth, and if they won't eat meaty bones, you may have to resort to this.

Homeopathic support for dental procedures

If your dog or cat needs a dental procedure, it is a very good idea to give the homeopathic remedy Arnica before and after, as this promotes healing of the gums, and noticeably reduces bleeding and soreness. Give a single dose of Arnica 30C the day before, repeat on the morning of the procedure, and follow up with two or more daily doses until all soreness has receded (typically only a day or two).

See more about administering homeopathic medicines on page 119, and about the use of Arnica on pages 129 and 200.

Gingivitis

In dogs, gingivitis is generally associated with tooth decay and poor oral hygiene, which, in my view, is often connected to an inappropriate diet. Cats, on the other hand, suffer from unique conditions of the gums that are not related to plaque or tartar, but are really the result of an ill-directed immune response. This autoimmune response, in which the body turns on itself, can lead to resorption of the roots of the teeth. In other cases, a red, inflamed line can be seen where the gums meet the teeth, although the teeth in themselves are completely healthy. This reaction can become very painful for the cat and lead to salivation and weight loss due to difficulty eating. Immunosuppressive drugs may help for a while, but sometimes only extraction of all of the teeth (even when the teeth are strong and healthy!) gives the cat relief.

As with all diseases of the immune

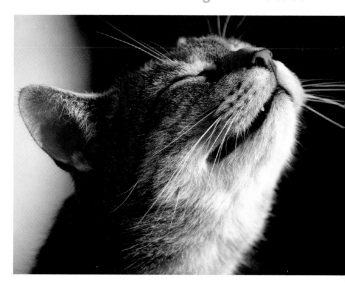

system, in my opinion holistic treatments such as acupuncture and homeopathy have a huge role to play. I can only hope that no cat owner will allow the extraction of a full mouth of healthy teeth without having exhausted all other treatment options.

DIARRHOEA AND VOMITING

Diarrhoea and vomiting are symptoms, not diseases. They may appear together or separately, and can be signs of either a serious illness or a harmless gut inflammation, perhaps after an animal has scavenged

Home management of simple acute diarrhoea

- *Always ensure access to fresh drinking water*
- *Enforce fasting for 24 hours (only for adult and otherwise healthy dogs)*
- *Give a probiotic supplement (for acute diarrhoea: a gel in a tube works well)*
- *Next, feed a digestible diet, little and often*
- *Always consult your vet if your animal becomes weak, if the stools contain blood or if the diarrhoea continues beyond a few days*

something that would have been best left alone.

Acute diarrhoea

In many cases, acute diarrhoea can be dealt with at home, but if your dog or cat becomes depressed or seems generally unwell, do take him to a vet straight away. The biggest immediate risk is dehydration, which shows as weakness. The risk of dehydration increases if there is also vomiting.

Provided, however, we are talking about an adult and otherwise healthy individual who remains bright and alert, with no sign of blood in the stools, most cases of acute diarrhoea can be safely managed at home in the following way.

Enforce a complete fast for up to 24 hours. Whether or not your dog is hungry, complete digestive rest will allow the gut lining to heal. Always provide free access to drinking water, but offer nothing else for 24 hours. After the day of fasting, offer an easily digestible bland diet in three to four small portions per day. The usual diet can be re-introduced gradually once the stools have returned to normal. Sometimes, you may get the same result by skipping the fast and moving directly to a bland diet, including a supplement containing probiotics together with a binding agent. See the section on supplements on page 213.

A digestible diet for cats

An easily digestible diet for cats should be low in carbohydrate, which means that dry foods are out. You want to feed a high-protein and high-liquid diet. This could be pure meat, tinned special diets or small amounts of normal tinned cat food. Some cat owners buy small jars of meat-based baby food for these situations. If you choose this option, make sure the product doesn't contain onion or artificial sweetener.

You can buy tinned special diets from your vet, or you can prepare a bland, meat-based diet at home.

As always when feeding cats, remember that the main thing is that they *do* eat (rather than *what* they eat). Where cats are concerned, menu suggestions are just that. At the end of the day, they get what they will eat.

The main principle involved here is that cats are poor at digesting carbohydrate, so, when possible, avoid feeding dry food or other sources of carbohydrate until their digestion has recovered.

If your cat has free outdoor access, consider keeping him indoors until you are satisfied that he is fully recovered. This way, you can be sure to see his stools so that you can monitor his symptoms, and avoid the risk of him deteriorating and deciding, as cats are prone to do, not to come home, but to hide away somewhere until he feels better.

A digestible diet for dogs

An easily digestible diet for a dog should be low in fat. Boiled white rice or mashed potatoes with some added cooked fish or chicken is a classic gentle diet for dogs. Feed about two thirds carbohydrate (potato or rice), and one third lean meat or fish. Don't add any fats. Do add a quality probiotic product (see below): these are readily available over the counter from your veterinary clinic.

Probiotics

The role of the microbiome (the microorganisms that live in the digestive tract) in maintaining gut health is a booming field in human as well as in veterinary medicine.

Probiotics are the naturally occurring beneficial gut bacteria. They can also be given as a supplement to rebalance the microbiome. Huge advances are expected in this area, and it is likely that pro- and prebiotics will usurp the role of antibiotics as research in this field leads to further discoveries.

The possibilities of improving health

by changing the bacterial gut flora goes far beyond treating digestive issues. Time will tell. Let me just say here that, for any acute or chronic digestive problem, the use of probiotics is among the very first steps to be taken. In the case of acute diarrhoea, there are several products that combine gut-restoring probiotics with a binding agent.

Probiotics are typically given as pills or powders, but, for acute cases, a tube of probiotic gel is often the preferred approach.

If your dog tends to scavenge and has regular stomach upsets as a result, it is worth keeping this in the house for first-line treatment, together with the steps described above.

Homeopathic treatment of acute diarrhoea
The homeopathic remedy Arsenicum album 30C suits a patient with acute-onset watery diarrhoea; perhaps with vomiting. If this matches your animal's symptom picture, try giving one dose every other hour. Another approach is to give a dose after each stool or vomit. This way, the dose frequency is automatically adjusted to the need, and you will give fewer doses as the patient improves.

Arsenicum album is probably the most commonly indicated homeopathic remedy in cases of acute diarrhoea, with or without vomiting. This is true whether the diarrhoea is caused by a bug or by your dog's scavenging of decayed matter. A dog eating a rotting crab found on the beach is a typical cause of this type of diarrhoea. See page 119 on giving homeopathic medicines.

There is a long list of other homeopathic remedies that suit other forms of diarrhoea. A few of these, with typical symptoms, are listed in the sidebar. Homeopathic remedies have no side effects. They work if the right remedy is chosen, but if you give a wrong remedy, nothing will happen. This means that experimentation is fine and can never do harm. Of course, always see your vet if

your animal seems ill from the diarrhoea, if he deteriorates and becomes weak, if the diarrhoea goes on beyond a few days, or if it contains blood.

Give a single dose every other hour or after each episode of stool or vomiting. If you haven't seen a clear response to the treatment after one day, don't continue the same remedy. In an acute situation, the correct remedy given as described above will work within a day.

Homeopathic treatment for acute diarrhoea

- *Watery diarrhoea with or without vomiting. The patients feels trembly and cold. Food poisoning. Desire for small sips of water, which may bring on vomiting:* Arsenicum album

- *Soft, mushy stools:* Podophyllum

- *Soft, mushy stools passed with an audible amount of wind:* Aloe

- *Yellow diarrhoea that may be particularly stinky. The patient feels hot, and will look for a cool place to lie down:* Sulphur

- *Stomach upset caused by overeating. Suits the animal who has gained access to the dinner table, the bin or food storage, and suffers the consequences:* Nux vomica (Nux vom)

- *Diarrhoea brought on by stress, especially the stress of being away from home. Suits the animal in a shelter or kennel, or the puppy or kitten who develops diarrhoea when brought to a new home:* Capsicum

Chronic diarrhoea
Chronic (constant or recurring) diarrhoea can result from a range of problems, which is as true for dogs and cats as it is for humans. It is always important to try to make the correct

diagnosis, which may involve endoscopy, scans or X-rays, as well as analysis of blood and stool samples.

There is a range of relatively common disorders, characterised by chronic inflammation of the digestive tract, that are collectively labelled inflammatory bowel disease (commonly referred to as IBD). IBD is a relatively common cause of chronic diarrhoea in both dogs and cats, and is believed to be caused by an overreacting and imbalanced immune system. The conventional treatment relies on ongoing symptomatic treatment with immune-modulating drugs, very much like the treatments used to treat allergic skin disease (see page 148 on the general mechanisms behind the treatment of allergic and autoimmune disease).

A diagnosis of IBD can be made based on the symptoms and exclusion of other causes of diarrhoea. It can be confirmed by taking a biopsy of the intestine and finding immune cells in the intestinal wall. This is a fairly invasive test and not without risk. In many cases, it is not absolutely needed to reach a diagnosis.

Treatment of inflammatory bowel disease

The conventional treatment of IBD relies on ongoing symptomatic treatment with immune-modulating drugs. Because of the risk of serious side effects associated with long-term use of these, other solutions should always be explored.

As described on page 149, imbalances of the immune system, like IBD, are, in my experience, best treated with holistic treatments such as TCM acupuncture or individualised classical homeopathy. In many cases, these treatments will be able to bring about a complete cure. Supplements such as slippery elm tree bark and psyllium husks form a protective layer that soothes the intestinal wall, and can be very helpful until a more permanent cure has been reached.

Constipation

Be aware that constipation can easily be confused with obstruction of the urethra, which is a much more serious problem. If your dog or cat is restless and constantly squatting and straining, they may be having trouble passing urine rather than stool. While constipation is rarely an emergency, urinary obstruction is one of the few truly life-threatening emergencies for which treatment cannot be delayed, even for a few hours.
If in doubt, always consult a vet immediately.

CONSTIPATION

Constipation (infrequent or difficult bowel movements) can occur for multiple reasons ranging from dietary problems to dehydration or intestinal disease.

Constipation doesn't tend to be a big problem in dogs. Conditions such as an enlarged prostate or blocked anal sacs can make bowel movements painful or difficult, however, so always consult a vet if your dog is having problems pooing. Changes in diet, such as the feeding of bone, can cause temporary constipation. As long as your dog isn't vomiting, remains bright and alert, and the constipation lasts no more than a day or two, there is rarely a need for further action.

Many cats, on the other hand, suffer from a chronic tendency to constipation, and it is important to see a vet, to both provide relief for your cat and try to find the root of the problem, and make the changes needed in time to prevent permanent damage to the large intestine.

The root of the problem can be many and varied –

- Long-haired cats may suffer from hairballs
- Some cats avoid using the litter tray

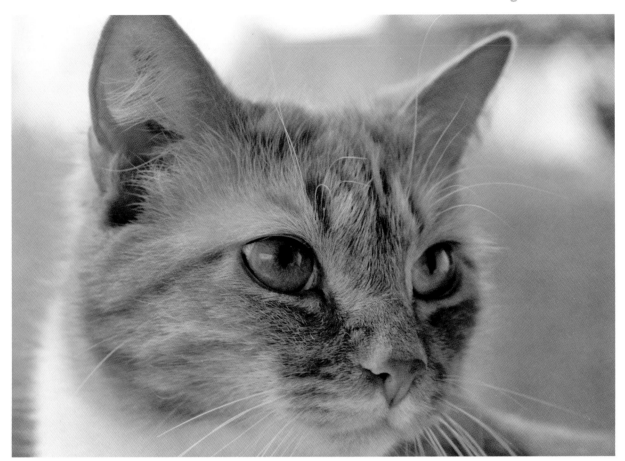

because they dislike where it is placed or the litter being used

- There may be too few trays in a multi-cat household, or perhaps a very fastidious cat doesn't find the tray clean enough and prefers to hold it in
- Old or overweight cats can suffer from loss of intestinal mobility
- Dehydration is another common cause of constipation

As discussed in the chapter on feeding (see page 25), cats fed primarily on dry kibble will be permanently slightly dehydrated, even when fresh water is available and they seem to be drinking fine. Many older cats suffer from kidney disease: another common cause of dehydration (see page 184).

Megacolon is a condition seen in cats, where long-term constipation has caused irreparable damage to the wall of the large intestine, which becomes dilated and no longer able to contract. Normal intestinal mobility cannot be restored, and the cat will need careful management for the rest of his life. In some cases, megacolon is found without a prior history of long-term constipation. The reason for this is unknown, but it is believed to be a hereditary problem. Megacolon, then, can be both a reason for and a consequence of chronic constipation.

Treating constipation

Naturally, the first step is to establish the cause of the problem. In cases where constipation is secondary to physical illness, this must be diagnosed and treated. When constipation is caused by behavioural issues, these must be identified and the necessary changes made to the environment. Some cases of recurring constipation are cured by simply making sure that the cat has his own litter tray that is placed in a calm and private spot, and cleaned after each visit.

Longhaired cats may need more frequent brushing and regular doses of one of the hairball gels or pastes that aid passing of hair through the intestines.

Cats who obsessively over-groom and suffer constipation because of the hairs they ingest need further attention. This may be an allergic problem where the grooming is addressing an itch, or it may be a purely stress-related response. See more about over-grooming in cats on page 164.

There is some debate about the best way to feed a cat with a tendency to constipation. Some would say that added fibre is the way to go, and recommend special high-fibre diets, while others believe that dry food is part of the problem and should be completely avoided in cats with constipation.

My approach is to focus primarily on hydration. It does not make sense to me to feed a constipated animal dehydrated food (even if it is high in fibre), so my advice is to stop all dry food and, instead, feed only tinned cat food or fresh meat. If extra fibre is needed, a teaspoon of psyllium husks or another dietary-fibre supplement can easily be mixed into tinned cat food or minced meat.

For some cats, the above changes may not be enough. Cats who have developed megacolon and therefore have permanently decreased intestinal motility may need regular dosing with lactulose, which passes undigested through the digestive tract, drawing water into the intestines. Lifelong treatment with drugs to improve intestinal motility may be needed in severe cases, and blockages may need to be removed manually by a veterinary surgeon, with or without anaesthesia. Fluid therapy and enemas administered by your vet may also be needed when blockages occur.

Whatever the reason behind your cat's constipation, it always makes sense to avoid dry food and try to increase his water intake. Good hydration will always help, regardless of whether dehydration is caused by disease or because cats never drink enough. See more about encouraging cats to drink in the chapter on urinary problems on page 181.

Together with the steps described above, acupuncture and homeopathy may be able to improve digestion, and can make a difference in some cases.

Osteopathy is always worthwhile for cats with a tendency to constipation. Whether the problem is caused by or has resulted in tension in the pelvic area, osteopathy can help.

Anal sacs

Unlike humans, but like other carnivorous mammals, dogs and cats have anal sacs: small, paired scent glands located on each side of the rectum.

The lining of the sacs contain glands that produce a dark liquid, which can only be described as the stinkiest substance in the world. This substance is emptied into the rectum through ducts that lead to the inner edge of the anus.

When a stool is passed, it squeezes the sacs so that a few drops of the stinky stuff are expressed to coat the stool. This is the reason behind all the bum and poo sniffing going on in the dog world. The anal sac fluid is how each dog leaves his own unique, scent-based visiting card.

In most dogs and cats, this system works impeccably, and there is no need for you (or your groomer or vet) to go anywhere near the anal sacs. You don't even need to know that they exist. It is a common misconception that 'checking' or expressing the anal glands is a part of good grooming or healthcare; not so. If there is no reason to suspect problems, please don't touch them.

It happens occasionally – much more commonly in dogs than in cats – that the sacs, for whatever reason, don't empty properly. If the sacs become over-filled and blocked, the dog will feel acutely uncomfortable, and will typically scoot on the floor or spin around to lick his bum. If you see this behaviour, take him to your vet. She will examine the anal sacs and, if they are not painful or blocked, and no other reason can be found, probably ask for a fresh stool sample to check for worms, the other main cause of dogs scooting on or licking their rear ends. (If your dog poos before you go to the vet, take along the sample.)

If the anal sacs are impacted and sore, the vet can generally express them quickly and easily, which will bring your dog immediate and immense relief. While it is important, of course, that this is done to relieve a deeply uncomfortable dog, it is equally important not to touch the sacs unless there is a reason to do so. Every time the anal sacs are manually expressed, it inflames them, which can lead to a vicious circle of inflamed and over-producing sacs that come to need regular manual emptying. This contributes to further inflammation, and eventually the natural balance is completely compromised and the sacs no longer empty into the rectum with each stool.

If the impaction and constant inflammation of the sacs leads to infection, the condition becomes acutely painful and requires antibiotic treatment. In some cases, an abscess forms, and it is necessary to clean and flush the area under general anaesthesia. Some dogs end up with anal sacs so scarred and destroyed that they are surgically removed. This is quite a complicated surgical procedure that carries a small risk of permanent faecal incontinence due to damage to the anal sphincter; a situation that could have been avoided.

Multiple theories exist about why some dogs suffer so badly from inflamed anal sacs whilst others never feel a thing, and many owners are completely unaware of their existence, as they cause no symptoms at all.

One theory is that inflamed anal sacs, much like inflamed ears, may be an expression of an underlying allergic problem. Others blame a tendency to soft stools as the main problem for most of these dogs. If the stools are too soft to express the sacs as they pass through the rectum (whether during a brief period of diarrhoea or over a longer term), the secretions will accumulate, and problems may follow. Seeing how crumbly-hard the stools become when dogs are fed a more natural diet of raw meat and bones, it is easy to suspect that our highly processed and mainly carbohydrate-based dog foods, when they pass through the dog, are simply too soft to work as nature intended.

Treating anal sac problems

In an acute situation, relieving the pressure by emptying the sacs is the important thing. If infection is present, your vet will probably also recommend antibiotic treatment, as either a cream, tablets, or both.

It can sometimes be tricky to get the sacs to empty naturally again following an impaction or infection. Once the sacs are inflamed, they definitely tend to overproduce, starting a vicious circle of inflammation that necessitates intervention, that adds to the inflammation … and on it goes. Previous infections may have caused scarring and a narrowing of the ducts that empty into the rectum, making it hard to get back on track. Some dogs, having experienced pain, may become more reluctant and cautious in their toilet habits. It may simply be that whatever caused the first case of impaction has not been resolved. In any case, anal sac problems often become chronic, and recur once something has gone wrong.

If you find yourself in this situation, there are several steps you can take before resorting to having the sacs surgically removed, a procedure that should be regarded as the absolute last option.

The most obvious step is to change the diet. Prevention is always easier than cure, but even if you already face chronic anal sac problems, it is still worth seeing what can be achieved through a simple diet change. There are two reasons for this. Firm stools are a prerequisite for proper anal sac function, and no one has firmer stools than the dog on a raw meat and bone diet. Secondly, if your dog suffers from an allergy (whether to storage mites in dry food or to certain foods), a diet change can address this.

Homeopathy and acupuncture are both excellent at treating chronic inflammation, and can make a real difference in cases of chronic anal sac problems.

Osteopathy can address tensions or imbalances in the pelvic area that may have caused the problem in the first place, and are certainly likely to be present after one or more painful episodes. An osteopathic assessment is therefore always a good idea for any dog who has suffered more than one episode of blocked anal sacs.

Leave them sacs alone

It is easy to be overzealous, potentially creating a problem that wasn't there to begin with. The anal sacs don't need manual emptying just because they are half-full. They don't have to be empty. They have a job to do, and generally do it best when we don't interfere. If the sacs are bulging, inflamed and painful, by all means get them expressed by a vet. If not, leave them alone

HEART AND AIRWAYS

KENNEL COUGH

Kennel cough is not one disease but a lumping together of many different causes of acute upper-airway symptoms in dogs. The correct term, canine infectious respiratory disease complex, is just much less catchy, so kennel cough it is.

Kennel cough is nothing more than the canine equivalent of the common cold. Your dog may have a snotty nose, and the most common symptom is a deep, dry cough that worsens with excitement or activity. The disease is very infectious but generally harmless, and it doesn't require specific treatment, except in the very weak or elderly.

Symptoms will generally clear after a couple of weeks of coughing, with or without symptomatic treatment.

Treatment of kennel cough

Remember that this is nothing more than a cold or a sore throat. An adult and otherwise healthy dog will generally recover in a few weeks without treatment. This is a very infectious condition, however, so your dog should be kept away from other dogs to prevent the infection spreading.

Let him rest until completely recovered. Light exercise is okay, but he should not be working or be allowed to play rough or be too active. If he pulls on the lead and the collar makes him cough, it is a good idea to use a harness instead. Sometimes, breathing in moisture can bring relief from the dry cough: it may help to have your dog stay in the bathroom when you shower.

Just like when humans get a cold or case of tonsillitis, all anyone can do is rest, try not to pass on the infection, and wait for it to go.

If your dog develops a high temperature,

the cough becomes productive, or he becomes very affected by the infection and loses his appetite and joie de vivre, do take him to the vet and have him checked.

Complications such as pneumonia can occur, especially in dogs who are already weakened by chronic illness, and in the very young and very old.

Prevention of kennel cough
The most important preventative step is to isolate sick dogs until the infection has passed.

Vaccination
A vaccine is available, and many vets still recommend annual vaccination against kennel cough. The World Small Animal Veterinary Association (WSAVA) has classified this as a non-core vaccine, meaning that it is not recommended for routine use in all dogs.

Furthermore, several experts are adamant that the vaccine is so ineffective and the disease so harmless that routine vaccination against kennel cough makes little sense.

See the chapter on vaccination on page 55 for further information.

Homeopathic nosodes
If you are aware of kennel cough in your dog's social circle – maybe some of his usual playmates are coughing or your dog trainer reports that the infection is around – I recommend giving the homeopathic kennel-cough nosode (Kennel Cough 30C) once daily for several weeks.

In my opinion this is a classic example of a situation in which nosodes can be very effective. As discussed earlier, I do not support regular preventative dosing with nosode mixes as a substitute for real vaccines, but daily dosing with a single nosode in the face of known exposure is a different matter entirely.

VIRAL DISEASE IN CATS

Cat flu
Cat flu is probably the most common infectious disease in cats: a highly infectious and potentially quite serious infection of the airways. The two most important causes of cat flu (feline infectious upper respiratory disease) are herpesvirus and calicivirus. Both of these are core vaccines in cats, meaning that WSAVA recommends regular vaccination of all cats against flu. See page 57 on the recommended use of cat flu vaccination.

Cat flu spreads quickly among the local cat population, causing much coughing and spluttering. Cats suffering from acute infection will be feverish. The eyes, nose and mouth can all be affected. Sick cats will stop eating, and some will develop pneumonia. Most adult cats will survive, although some will be unable to eliminate the virus, and may suffer from chronic cat flu or become healthy carriers of infection.

Other causes of viral disease in cats
Several serious viral diseases are widespread among cats. Apart from cat flu, FeLV (feline leukaemia) and FIV (feline Aids) are common in many areas, particularly among free-roaming cats. See page 89 for a discussion of the best ways to protect your cat against these infections.

The severity of disease in individual cats varies enormously. Sometimes, a cat is so ill at the time of diagnosis that the vet will recommend euthanasia. In other cases, a diagnosis is made in a cat who shows only mild symptoms, or has no symptoms at all. In many of these cases, the cat can live with the infection for a long time. Your vet will be able to advise you on steps to take to avoid infecting other cats.

It may be worth mentioning that none of the cat viruses can infect people.

Treatment of chronic viral infections in cats

Cats who are diagnosed with chronic viral infections are likely to need regular veterinary care, depending on the degree and nature of their symptoms. These chronic viral infections are not considered curable, but correct symptomatic treatment is important.

For instance, because these cats have compromised immune systems, they are susceptible to secondary infections that may require antibiotic treatment. This is true in the case of chronic cat flu as well as for other cat viruses. Many cats, in fact, suffer concurrently from more than one viral infection.

Apart from the above supportive conventional treatment from your vet, a lot can be done to strengthen your cat and support his immune system to generally improve his quality of life, and ensure maximum resistance to complications. Providing a high-quality diet, minimising the use of toxins and ensuring a stress-free environment are all steps you can take that can make a big difference. Also, I cannot over-emphasise the benefit I see when treating these cats with deep-acting, individualised homeopathic treatment.

ASTHMA

Asthma is relatively common in cats; the result of an allergic reaction to inhaled allergens. See page 148 for more information about allergies. In some cases, the symptoms are affected by seasonal changes. Smoking in the home will exacerbate a cat's asthma. Some cats react to certain types of cat litter. Overall, however, the cause of the symptoms is difficult or even impossible to identify.

The main symptom is a chronic cough. In serious cases, there may be episodes where the cat struggles to breathe. The forced exhalation will be audible, and the cat will sit hunched up, breathing through an open mouth. This situation requires immediate veterinary attention.

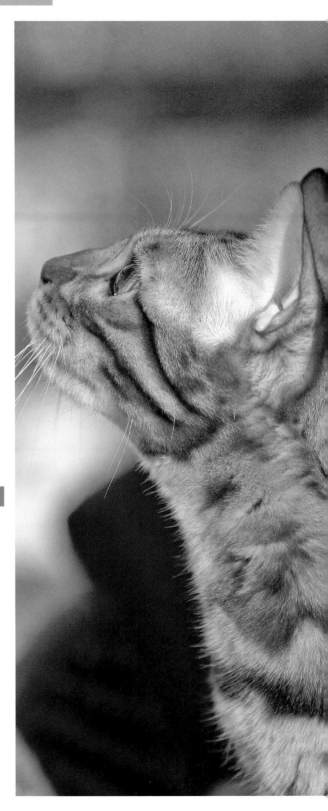

Treatment of asthma

It is important that your vet monitors the patient regularly. Experimenting at home with antihistamines or cough medicine is **not** recommended. Antibiotics are rarely needed, unless the condition is complicated by infection. Some cats need long-term treatment with steroids, which are typically administered every other day to minimise side effects. In many cases, medicine administered through an inhaler (rather than in tablet form or as injections) is tolerated well.

As in all allergic conditions, deep-acting treatment with homeopathy or acupuncture is invaluable. It is crucial that this treatment is in the hands of a vet, though, as we are talking about a potentially life-threatening disease.

HEART DISEASE

Heart disease is commonly diagnosed in both cats and dogs. Some breeds are predisposed to certain heart problems.

Heart disease should always be diagnosed and treated by a specialist veterinary cardiologist. It is not always possible to diagnose heart disease correctly by merely listening to the heart through a stethoscope. Some heart murmurs turn out to be of no consequence. If your vet hears a murmur during a routine health check, you will typically be referred to a specialist for a full diagnosis, which is likely to include an ultrasound scan.

I will limit my discussion of this topic to the following list of supplements that are often helpful in animals suffering from heart disease.

- Fish oils (essential fatty-acid supplementation)
- Coenzyme Q10
- Crataegus (herbal or homeopathic)
- Amino-acid supplementation (specifically carnitine and cysteine)

Individualised treatment in the hands of an experienced veterinary herbalist, homeopath or acupuncturist can strengthen the function of the heart, as well as the patient as a whole.

Heart disease is not an area that lends itself to home treatment. The above is intended simply as an illustration of the fact that, even in the case of serious illness, there are supplements and treatments that can be beneficial as an adjunct to conventional treatment, and which may even mean the difference between life and death.

THYROID DISEASE

Thyroid disease is very common in both dogs and cats. The thyroid glands tend to under-function in dogs (hypothyroidism), while many cats suffer from overactivity of the thyroid (hyperthyroidism).

Conventional treatment of thyroid disease

Both conditions (decreased levels of thyroid hormones in dogs and increased levels in cats) are most commonly treated for the rest of the animal's life with daily medication given at home.

For hyperthyroid cats, other conventional treatment options are available. In some cases, indoor cats can be managed simply by feeding a special iodine-free diet. Surgery to remove the thyroid glands is also an option, and, finally, hyperthyroid cats can be admitted to a special facility for treatment with radioactive iodine that destroys the thyroid tissue. The cat must stay in the facility for one to four weeks, until he is no longer radioactive, for environmental and human health and safety reasons.

Holistic treatment of thyroid disease

It is my clear personal experience that hypothyroid dogs can, in most cases, be completely cured through holistic treatment. Find a vet who can prescribe individualised homeopathic treatment or a vet trained in traditional Chinese medicine. Both treatment modalities are obvious choices in this situation: find the one that works for your dog.

When it comes to cats with hyperthyroidism, the clinical picture varies enormously depending on the cat's age, how advanced the disease is, whether the cat also suffers from other illnesses, and so on. Sufferers are typically elderly cats, and many also have some degree of compromised kidney function.

This may not be diagnosed until the body's own method of increasing kidney output – 'turning up the pressure' by developing hyperthyroidism – is removed through treatment, meaning that kidney disease is then exposed. It is not uncommon for kidney disease to be diagnosed shortly after a cat begins treatment for hyperthyroidism, simply because one condition was masking the other. This is a good argument for treating hyperthyroid cats with medication for a while in order to assess the effect; even in cases where surgery or radioactive iodine treatment is planned.

It is crucial to support these elderly cats beyond simply treating their thyroid disease. Reducing stress, optimising diet, and taking care of their fluid balance are equally important areas to address. Many hyperthyroid cats benefit from homeopathic treatment. Some need a combination of holistic and conventional treatments to thrive, while others do fine on conventional or holistic treatment alone.

THE URINARY SYSTEM

The most common conditions affecting the lower urinary tract (urethra and bladder) are infection and inflammation (page 178), crystals or stones (page 182), and incontinence (page 183). Kidney disease is discussed on page 184.

CYSTITIS

Anyone can suffer a simple bout of cystitis, and dogs and cats who are diabetic or being treated with steroids are at increased risk of developing cystitis. If the same individual gets cystitis repeatedly, the underlying problem must be addressed.

The first sign of cystitis in dogs may just be a lot of rear-end licking. Sometimes there is frequent urination or even blood in the urine. In cats, often the only sign is urination outside of the litter box. Sudden peeing on the floor in an otherwise house-trained animal can also be a tell-tale sign of cystitis in dogs.

There is a risk of misinterpreting this as a behavioural problem. If you suspect cystitis, it's a good idea to take a fresh urine sample when you take your dog or cat to the vet. This is easier said than done, I know, but a strategically-placed frying pan will often capture a few precious drops from a peeing dog. For cats, you can get cat litter designed for this purpose from your vet prior to the visit. Your vet can also relatively simply collect a sterile urine sample directly from your dog or cat's bladder.

Cystitis in dogs

Your vet will examine your dog as well as analyse a urine sample and possibly a blood sample. It is important to begin appropriate antibiotic treatment without delay. Let your vet check another urine sample at the end of the course of antibiotics to make sure that the infection is indeed completely gone.

In dogs, there is a tendency for mineral crystals to form around clusters of bacteria in the urine. This means that untreated or inadequately treated cystitis can lead to the formation of bladder stones.

If an otherwise healthy dog suffers from cystitis again and again, the problem warrants closer investigation. Blood and urine analysis, X-rays and scans are all useful steps to find the root of the problem. There may be an underlying undiagnosed systemic illness, or a local problem in the urinary tract that must be found or ruled out, such as stones, crystals, tumours, polyps, anatomical abnormalities or other causes.

If your dog develops cystitis for a second time, the antibiotic treatment must be based on careful examination of a urine sample, including urine culture and sensitivity testing. It is also a good idea to check a fresh urine sample a couple of weeks after the conclusion of antibiotic treatment.

The point here is that a simple bout of cystitis can happen to anyone. Once properly treated, it is no great cause for concern, but if it recurs, make sure it is treated in a targeted way to avoid chronic infections, and that it is not a symptom of a bigger problem.

Holistic treatment of cystitis in dogs

If your dog has a tendency to develop cystitis, get him examined properly to check for underlying causes, and make sure, in the acute phase, that the infections are treated quickly and appropriately with targeted antibiotic treatment.

On top of this, there are several things you can do to support his recovery, and reduce the risk of repeated bladder infections. Drinking plenty of liquids will help to flush bacteria and crystals from the bladder. You may want to stop feeding dry food and change your dog's diet to one with more natural water content to ensure proper hydration.

Cranberries contain a substance that prevents bacteria from adhering to the bladder wall. Food supplements containing cranberry are also widely available, and adding one on a daily basis may help prevent recurring infections. Other supplements that strengthen the lining of the bladder wall – and therefore make it harder for bacteria to settle – are widely available and can, together with

adequate water intake, make all the difference in preventing repeated infections. See page 25 on hydration and page 212 for supplements to support the bladder.

Acupuncture or deep-acting classical homeopathy can strengthen the individual as a whole, and address the susceptibility at its core.

Cystitis in cats

Cystitis in cats, unlike cystitis in dogs and humans, is only very rarely an actual bacterial infection. A cat with cystitis will experience acute pain when trying to pee, and the bladder will certainly be inflamed, but, in up to 90% of cases, there will be no infection.

Consequently, it makes no sense at all to treat cystitis in cats with antibiotics unless a urine analysis has demonstrated the presence of bacteria, placing the cat in the small minority of feline cystitis cases that are bacterial bladder infections. The fact that, in the majority of cases there are no bacteria to eliminate, doesn't mean that the condition requires no treatment, however. In the acute phase, which is very painful for the cat, painkilling medications are needed.

It is also, of course, vital to have your cat examined to get a proper diagnosis to ensure that he is not, in fact, constipated or suffering from bladder stones or a blocked urethra, as these conditions can also cause a cat to go in and out of the litter box, straining and complaining.

Factors known to increase the risk of feline idiopathic cystitis

- *Lack of outdoor access*
- *Use of a litter tray*
- *Dry food*
- *Living in a multi-cat household*

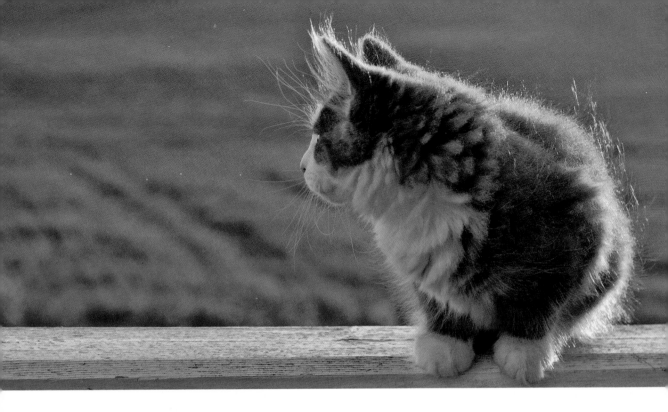

Why is peeing painful when there is no infection?

What is the reason for this common tendency in cats to develop an inflamed bladder and show all the signs of cystitis, but with no trace of bacterial infection?

The mechanisms are not completely understood, but it is believed that feline sterile cystitis (sterile because there is no infection) occurs as a response to stress. Cats are certainly easily stressed, and the two most common physical problems linked to stress are over-grooming and cystitis. See more about cats and stress on page 207.

It is likely that a combination of factors lead to the syndrome of feline sterile cystitis, also sometimes called feline idiopathic cystitis (idiopathic means that we see no reason for it; in this case because there is no bacterial infection).

When a cat experiences stress, the brain is affected, and, as a consequence, both the cat's behaviour and his perception of pain will be altered.

In the bladder, the natural defence mechanisms of the bladder wall will be weakened, making the mucosal lining of the bladder more susceptible to inflammation. Add to this the fact that, as described on page 25, cats have a very concentrated urine, even more so because of the problematic fluid balance associated with dry food. If a cat then takes against the litter tray for whatever reason, and consequently doesn't pee often enough, we are left with a wide range of contributory factors that need to be addressed to solve the problem.

Holistic treatment of cystitis in cats

The conventional veterinary surgeon cannot treat this condition beyond relieving the pain of acute flare-ups with painkilling medication, but that is not to say that nothing can be done about feline cystitis. This is absolutely a problem that can be treated – and cured. It takes a combined approach that addresses diet, fluid balance, lifestyle, and stress levels while strengthening the bladder wall specifically and, on a more general level, the resilience of the whole individual.

Behaviour is the key to this problem. Even if your cat has only suffered a single attack of idiopathic cystitis, you will need to take a close look at his lifestyle to try to identify possible stress factors. Maybe he is bored and needs more stimulation. Maybe he is frustrated by a lack of outdoor access. Maybe he doesn't get on with another cat in the household. Maybe he just needs spaces to hide away in and feel safe. Maybe he dislikes the litter tray, either because it is shared with other cats, is not in a safe and sheltered position, is not kept clean enough, or because he dislikes the type of litter being used.

While these issues are being identified and changes made, several measures can ease the perception of stress. A dietary supplement containing the amino acid tryptophan helps some cats feel calmer. The use of pheromones in the areas where the cat spends most of his time can have the same effect. See page 210.

Making his urine more dilute will lessen the irritation of the bladder wall. As described in the chapter on diet (page 24), cats have a very low thirst drive, and are often dehydrated

as a result, causing the urine to be more concentrated. This situation is made worse if the cat is fed dry food.

Improvements in the fluid balance can be made by changing to wet foods and by encouraging your cat to drink. Make sure the water bowl is in a safe and sheltered place, and not near the litter tray. Make sure the water is always fresh. Some cats dislike their whiskers touching the sides of the bowl, and will drink more if water is served in a wide, flat container. Many cats prefer running water, and

multi—pronged approach to curing recurring idiopathic cystitis in cats

- *Identify and change lifestyle stressors*
- *Avoid dry food and encourage drinking*
- *Use supplements to reduce the perception of stress and to strengthen the bladder lining*
- *Provide individualised classical homeopathy or acupuncture to strengthen the individual as a whole*

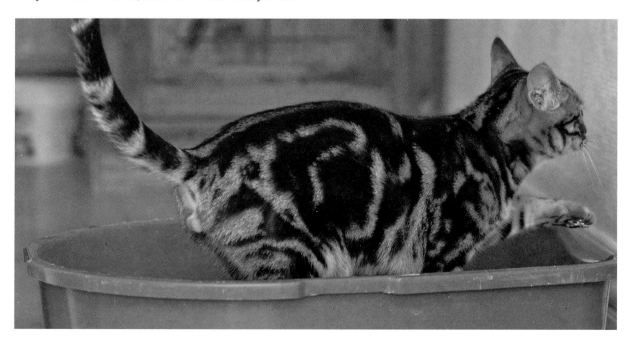

can be encouraged to drink by offering them water from a tap or cat fountain.

Another important area of focus is the bladder wall, the site of the inflammation that is causing pain. The mucosal lining of the bladder wall is further lined with a layer that protects against the corrosive effect of urine. We aim to strengthen this protective layer and repair any weakness or damage in order to preserve the integrity of the mucosal lining, and reduce inflammation. This protective layer is referred to as the GAG layer (GlycosAminoGlycan).

We can support the bladder wall by feeding supplements containing the building blocks needed to maintain the GAG layer: glucosamine, chondroitin, and hyaluronic acid.

Last, but certainly not least, deep-acting individual treatment with homeopathy or acupuncture can dramatically strengthen the cat, both physically and in the way he interacts with his surroundings, and to the stress of life.

URINARY CRYSTALS AND STONES

Urinary crystals form when minerals in the urine precipitate into crystals inside the bladder. These crystals may stick together and form larger stones, or may remain as a 'sludge' that is often referred to as 'sand' or 'gravel.'

Urinary crystals are a relatively common problem in both dogs and cats, and symptoms – and the course of the problem – depend on whether crystals occur in the form of sand or gravel rather than as discrete stones, and whether they are present primarily in the bladder or have become stuck in the urethra, causing an acute blockage.

The most common type of urinary crystal is struvite. Struvite crystals form when the urine pH is too alkaline, and are most commonly seen, at least in dogs, as a complication to bacterial bladder infections.

There are several other, more rarely seen, types of crystals. Some breeds are predisposed to crystal formation because of an inherited tendency to abnormal mineral metabolism.

Treatment of urinary crystals and stones

Traditionally, treatment consists of antibiotics for the bladder infections, and an attempt to dissolve urinary stones by normalising urine pH through the feeding of special diets. In the case of bladder stones too large to be passed naturally, surgical removal is the only alternative if dietary changes cannot dissolve the stones. It is important to continue checking the urine regularly for the presence of crystals, as about one third of patients go on to form new stones after surgery.

Opinions vary among veterinary experts about the wisdom of focusing entirely on identifying the crystals and monitoring and changing urinary pH. There is certainly a risk, when attempting to acidify the urine in order to dissolve struvite crystals, that the urine will become too acidic, and cause the opposite problem: formation of calcium oxalate crystals, which occur when urine pH becomes too low. This is why I cannot immediately support the many recommendations about natural ways to modify urine pH, such as feeding vitamin C, apple-cider vinegar, and so on.

A colleague once poetically compared urinary crystals in cats to autumn leaves on a garden path: the point being that they are not, in themselves, a problem. They are simply there as the result of a natural process. Problems arise only if they (leaves or crystals) are allowed to accumulate. Viewed in this way, it is not a problem in itself when urinary crystals are found in a urine sample. It only becomes a problem if build-up is allowed to occur, which happens when there is not enough urinary output to flush away the crystals (if the garden path is never swept clear of leaves).

See the discussion about fluid balance

in the diet chapter (page 24), and the advice on getting cats to drink more in the section on cystitis (page 179).

Encouraging a healthy fluid balance as a way to achieve a more dilute urine will solve many of the problems of the lower urinary tract. This is true whether we are talking about cystitis or crystal formation.

Just a thought ...

Maybe we could focus less on urinary pH levels and the presence or absence of urinary crystals if we ensure that our cats are properly hydrated, and that bladder infections in dogs are treated effectively

---

The blocked cat: a real emergency

Be aware that an animal who is unable to pass urine is suffering from one of the few genuinely life-threatening veterinary emergencies, and must be taken to the vet without delay.

Urinary obstruction happens when the urethra becomes blocked, trapping urine in the bladder. This is predominantly a problem seen in castrated male cats, as their urethra is very long and narrow, making obstruction much more likely to occur. If your cat keeps straining, or restlessly paces in and out of the litter tray, off to the vet he goes.

Treatment of urinary obstruction

The vet will empty the bladder, if possible by placing a urinary catheter. Once the pressure is relieved, the focus will be on establishing the reason and preventing recurrences. See the section earlier in this chapter (page 182) concerning urinary crystals.

Homeopathic support for a sore urethra

If your cat or dog has had a urinary catheter inserted, or has had surgery involving the bladder or urethra (such as removal of bladder stones or tumours), there are two homeopathic remedies you should know about, as these will aid his recovery. See more about homeopathic medicine on page 117.

First, give Calendula 30C twice daily for four to five days, followed by Staphysagria 200C once daily for three days. This will ensure optimal healing of the mucosal lining of the urethra, and/or bladder wall.

INCONTINENCE

Urinary incontinence is primarily a problem of neutered female dogs. As many as one in five female dogs develops this problem as a direct consequence of neutering, which is why the condition is often referred to as spay incontinence (the more correct term is acquired urethral sphincter mechanism incompetence).

The mechanism behind the problem is this: neutering removes the ovaries, which leads to a reduced level of circulating oestrogen in the body. Lack of oestrogen stimulation leads to decreased muscle tone of the bladder sphincter and urethra, and subsequently (in some dogs) to urine leakage. In most cases, incontinence starts two to three years after neutering, but can appear at any time, ranging from a few weeks after neutering to many years later.

The risk of developing spay incontinence increases with the size of the breed. It is most common in large and giant breeds and uncommon in small breeds (dogs weighing less than 15kg). It is one of the many health risks associated with neutering. While spay incontinence has been recognised for many years and remains the most common serious side effect of neutering, we are becoming increasingly aware, especially since 2013 see page 76), of many more far-reaching negative consequences of routine neutering of both males and females

This topic is covered on page 76.

Treatment of spay incontinence

As the cause of the problem was permanent removal of the ovaries, it follows that spay incontinence requires daily lifelong treatment.

Two groups of medication can be tried: synthetic oestrogen, and medication to increase urethral tone. If one approach doesn't solve the incontinence, the two medications may be tried together. Some bitches suffer side effects from long-term medication, and others become non-responsive to treatment, so that the incontinence recurs.

Although there is no guarantee that treatment will work or that it will remain safe or effective, many bitches do respond well to medication for many years, with their incontinence well controlled.

Holistic treatment of spay incontinence

Spay incontinence is high on my list of conditions for which holistic treatment is the way to go.

If your bitch is diagnosed with this problem, seek the help of a vet trained in traditional Chinese medicine or in classical homeopathy. It is my personal experience that homeopathy works better than conventional treatment for most of these patients. Even when conventional medication successfully controls the incontinence, finding a long-term solution without the risk of side effects is always worthwhile.

The homeopathic remedy Sepia 30C is effective in many cases of spay incontinence. Provided the diagnosis is clear, you may want to try giving it daily for a few weeks. If it doesn't stop the incontinence, see a veterinary homeopath for help in finding the correct individual remedy for your dog. See page 117 on homeopathic treatment of dogs.

CHRONIC KIDNEY DISEASE

There are many different causes of kidney disease in dogs and cats, so I will limit my discussion to chronic renal insufficiency ('kidney failure'); the common end stage of kidney disease.

Chronic kidney disease is one of the most common health problems in aging cats, but is less common in dogs. I therefore refer to cats, although the points made are equally relevant for dogs with chronic renal failure.

Chronic kidney disease is not a curable condition: once kidney cells have died, the tissue cannot regenerate. This doesn't mean, however, that nothing can be done for the patient with chronic irreversible kidney damage. Far from it. There are several steps you can take both to strengthen your cat in general, and to ensure that his kidney function remains as good as possible for as long as possible.

Kidney disease often goes undiagnosed until the majority of kidney function is lost, and physical symptoms become evident. The three main health consequences of deficient kidney function are a disturbed fluid balance, accumulation in the blood of waste products that are normally excreted by the kidneys (azotemia), and high levels of phosphate in the blood.

The first signs of kidney disease that most people notice in their animals are increased thirst and urination, reduced appetite, and weight loss. When the kidneys lose the ability to concentrate urine, the cat will pass an increased amount of dilute urine. As a consequence, he will drink more to try to make up for the lost fluid, but eventually he will become dehydrated.

Treatment of chronic renal failure

Kidney failure cannot be cured, but in many cases a cat can live with it without compromising his quality of life. I have known many cats (and dogs) with chronic renal failure who have lived active lives for years following the diagnosis. Your vet will probably prescribe medication to enhance kidney function, and possibly a supplement (phosphate binder) to control the level of phosphorus in the blood.

It is crucial that your cat has access to fresh drinking water at all times. Common-sense steps to prevent dehydration, such as avoiding dry foods and installing a water fountain, are discussed in the diet chapter (page 24), and in the sections on lower urinary tract disease (page 181). If your cat does become dehydrated, a few hours on a drip at the vet's can often get him back on his feet, and feeling (and therefore eating and drinking) better.

Your vet may also recommend regular injections of vitamin B and anabolic steroids to help your cat maintain his bodyweight.

On top of these measures, there are several useful supplements (primarily herbal) that can support kidney function.

Individualised treatment from a herbalist, a TCM acupuncturist or a classical homeopath can support the individual at a deep level, and make all the difference between steady decline and thriving, although no treatment will be able to permanently restore the kidneys.

What to feed a kidney patient

Confusion and controversy dominates the debate among vets when it comes to the question of limiting dietary protein in the face of kidney disease. I have yet to see any evidence that a high-protein diet puts strain on the kidneys or exacerbates kidney disease in any way.

At the very end stage of advanced kidney disease, when only minimal organ function remains, nitrogen waste products will accumulate in the blood and make the patient feel unwell. Human kidney patients describe nausea and tiredness as the main symptoms. At this stage of the disease, there may be some merit to limiting the intake of protein, simply to minimise waste products. Still, I do not believe that there is any sense to the often-quoted advice that kidney patients

should be fed a low-protein diet from the point of diagnosis. I repeat: no matter what you may hear, it is not possible to damage the kidneys by feeding 'too much' protein.

The most important point about diet and kidney disease is that it is much more important that the patient does eat, rather than what he eats. Your vet will no doubt suggest that you feed a proprietary kidney diet, designed to be calorie-dense and low in phosphate. If your cat is happy to eat this, by all means let him, although I strongly recommend sticking to the tinned version, as it makes little sense to feed dehydrated food to someone whose biggest health threat is dehydration.

However, if, as is often the case, your cat is not tempted by the kidney diet, let him eat whatever he fancies. Keeping him eating and maintaining his weight are the goals here. Don't get into battles you can't win by denying him what he likes because you think something else is better for him. Chances are,

HOMEMADE KIDNEY DIET

The American vet Jean Dodds recommends the following homemade diet for a late-stage kidney patient

- ⅔ boiled white rice or mashed potatoes
- ⅓ fish, pork or duck
- Blended vegetables may be added. Scrambled eggs can also be added if the patient can digest them

Feed small portions at least four times daily

If your cat won't eat

- *Feed little and often*
- *Don't leave food out. Remove any leftovers or untouched food*
- *Heating the food can make it much more appealing*
- *Junk food is better than no food*

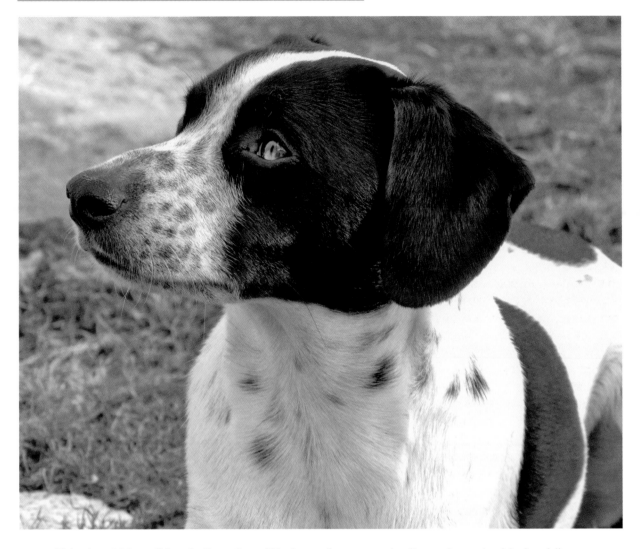

you will just put him off food altogether. Work with him – indeed, spoil him. If your vet just sold you a large bag of dry kidney diet but your cat will only eat grilled chicken in a cream sauce, I know whose side I'm on. There are many ways to increase calorie intake, and if he won't eat the veterinary low-phosphate diet, you can simply add a phosphate binder to the food that he will eat.

It is my personal opinion that force-feeding and long-term use of appetite-stimulating drugs have no place when it comes to the chronic renal patient. In some other situations, force-feeding *can* serve a purpose:

for example, it can be valuable in aiding recovery after surgery, or in other situations in which the patient needs short-term support until he is expected to recover and regain his appetite. When the patient is suffering chronic organ failure, however, the situation is a very different one, and force-feeding under these circumstances is an undignified intervention that I find ethically indefensible.

Spoil him, tempt him; follow the advice in this chapter in an effort to entice him. But if he really won't eat, that, to me, is a sign that he doesn't want to live any longer, and I believe that this should be respected.

THE REPRODUCTIVE SYSTEM

PYOMETRA

Pyometra (infection of the womb) is fairly commonly seen in elderly intact (unneutered) female dogs.

In some cases, there is a discharge from the vulva, and you may notice spots on the floor or in your dog's bedding. More commonly, a lot of rear-end licking is the only clue, and closely examining the vulva may then reveal a discharge.

In some cases there is no discharge (closed pyometra), which is why it is important to consider pyometra whenever an intact bitch seems off-colour; especially so during the first one to two months after her season, when the risk of pyometra is highest. Pyometra is a serious, even potentially life-threatening illness that requires immediate treatment.

Misalliance injections (an antiprogestagenic drug which is licenced for the prevention of unwanted pregnancy in bitches, sometimes given after accidental mating) involve an increased risk of pyometra.

If you have an intact bitch, be aware that there is a period of increased risk after each season, but it is safe to say that any dog with a womb can develop a womb infection. The symptoms may be very acute, requiring emergency treatment, or much less serious, causing a gradual onset of fatigue and lack of appetite. Many bitches with pyometra show an increased thirst. There will not always be a raised body temperature, just as not all cases will have a vaginal discharge.

What this means in practice is that if your bitch is off-colour, possibly drinking more than usual, get her checked out by your vet. Better safe than sorry.

You may still hear the old myth that a bitch who exhibits strong symptoms of false pregnancy has a higher risk of developing pyometra. This was once cited as a reason for neutering bitches with a tendency to false pregnancy, but the argument has no merit. The only connection between false pregnancy and pyometra is that only intact bitches get them. You can read more about false pregnancy on page 84. While false pregnancy is a natural state, pyometra is always a sign of serious illness that requires an immediate trip to the vet.

Treatment of pyometra

Pyometra is one of the few diseases that all dog owners must be aware of and know to look out for, as it can occur acutely and develop very quickly. This is not one of those situations where it is okay to leave it for a day or two, or try to treat it at home before seeking veterinary assistance.

The most effective treatment for pyometra is surgical removal of the womb. In some cases, it may be safe to treat this condition medically to preserve the womb, but recurrences are common, and the treatment will have to be followed closely by your vet.

If your bitch has a mild case of open pyometra that your vet is happy to treat conservatively (with medication rather than surgery), I strongly recommend that you support this treatment with acupuncture or homeopathy. These treatments have a profound effect on the womb, and may reduce the risk of recurrence and other complications. If, however, your vet feels that immediate surgery is the only safe way to go, this is not worth risking your dog's life for. Get it done.

If your bitch is having surgery for pyometra, give the homeopathic remedy Arnica as described on page 200. Furthermore, I recommend giving a daily dose of Sepia 200C for three days about two weeks after the surgery.

CRYPTORCHIDISM

The testicles are formed in the abdomen and

descend during normal foetal development through the inguinal canal into the scrotal sacs. If, for whatever reason, this process doesn't happen, one or both testicles may remain either in the abdomen or in the inguinal canal.

If one or both testicles are not in the scrotum when the puppy or kitten is six to eight weeks old, the animal is said to be cryptorchid. In a few cases, the testicle(s) descend as late as six months after birth, but generally speaking they are not expected to descend if they have not already done so by the age of two months.

The standard advice is that a cryptorchid dog should be castrated, partly because a retained testicle has a higher risk of developing cancer than one in the scrotum, and partly because cryptorchidism is an inherited tendency, so the animal should not be allowed to breed. Castrating a cryptorchid male involves more complicated surgery than a standard castration, depending on where the retained testicle(s) are to be found.

The cryptorchid male is in no way affected by his condition. The reason for surgery is the increased cancer risk. Opinions vary, but some sources cite the risk as being 16 times higher than for a normal testicle. Admittedly, this isn't quite as bad as it may sound, as testicular cancer is treatable, and only rarely fatal. Remember, though, that the retained testicle is out of sight and so cannot be examined, meaning that a cancer (which would be easily noticed as a lump on a normal testicle in the scrotum) would not be discovered.

If your dog is cryptorchid on one side and you are not planning on having him castrated, you may choose to have only the retained testicle removed, and have a vasectomy done on the normal side. This way, you can take all of the responsible steps (no increased cancer risk and no risk of passing on the trait) but have a hormonally intact dog.

This condition is less common in cats, and, as most male cats are castrated anyway, it will have been dealt with.

THE NERVOUS SYSTEM

SEIZURES

Seizures occur as a result of uninhibited chaotic firing of signals in the brain. If your animal suffers a seizure that lasts more than two minutes, or if he has several seizures on the same day, it is a potentially life-threatening emergency, and he should be taken straight to the vet. An isolated seizure, on the other hand, is not nearly as serious as it is frightening to observe. If your dog or cat has a single seizure, this is not a great emergency. It is fine to make an appointment to see the vet in a few days.

A seizure can happen anywhere, at any time, but most seizures happen from sleep. If your animal is at the top of a staircase or in another position where he may fall or in other ways hurt himself, you may have no choice but to move him. If it is safe to do so, however, it is best to leave him be during the seizure.

It is tempting to want to comfort him, stroke him or reassure him with your voice, but this is not a good idea. This is partly because you may get hurt but also because the best thing to do for him is to reduce sensory input, not add to it. So, don't call out to the rest of the family, don't say his name, and don't touch him at all. Step away, turn off the TV or radio, and dim the lights. Simply stay calm and give him space.

You may want to time or film the seizure: you can be certain that your vet will ask how long it lasted. When your dog or cat comes to, he will be disoriented and confused. Again, give him space. Most will appreciate a meal once they have recovered, and may then be ready for a rest. Within a surprisingly short time, it will be as though it never happened.

EPILEPSY

A seizure is not an illness, it is a symptom. Poisoning, brain damage, liver disease, kidney disease, infection, diabetes, and tumours are just some of the problems that can cause seizures.

When you take your animal to the vet after the first seizure(s), her initial job is twofold: to look for a reason for the seizure(s), and to assess whether the seizure(s) are so serious as to warrant treatment.

In the majority of cases in which dogs and cats have repeated seizures, we are not able to find anything wrong at all. Typically, urine and blood samples will be taken (to rule out some of the potential reasons for seizures listed above), and sometimes a brain scan will be performed. When, as tends to be the case, the results come back normal, the patient is given the diagnosis 'idiopathic epilepsy,' which simply means 'seizures for no known reason.'

Keep a log of dates and times of seizures. This makes it much easier to assess over time whether the epilepsy is under control or whether the intervals are getting shorter and the seizures getting longer. It also helps identify any patterns or triggers. Perhaps the intervals are fixed, or maybe the seizures consistently happen when your animal is exposed to certain activities or treatments.

Also, consider any exposure or changes your animal may have experienced in the period just before the first seizure. At the very least, this information will be valuable to the homeopath or acupuncturist who is trying to help your dog or cat overcome this problem.

Be aware that some of the oral treatments available to protect against fleas and ticks may cause seizures, and that these drugs are to be avoided in any animal who has ever had a seizure. Personally, I prefer to avoid their use in any animal.

Some breeds or lines are predisposed to epilepsy. It goes without saying that an animal with epilepsy should not be used for breeding.

Treatment of epilepsy

The standard treatment of epilepsy is daily medication to prevent seizures. This is only recommended when the seizures are relatively frequent, unusually long-lasting, or tend to happen in clusters. If your animal has a fit every three to four months, he will generally not be put on medication.

If medication is started, the aim is not to stop the seizures completely, but to reduce the severity and frequency of seizures without too many side effects.

It is important to monitor the patient regularly. Typically, a full physical examination, including blood tests, will be done two to four times per year to ensure that the medication is being optimally dosed, and is still tolerated by the patient. Medication, when effective, will be lifelong.

Holistic treatment of epilepsy

Holistic treatment of epilepsy is, perhaps, most relevant in cases where standard medications are not effective at controlling seizures, or are associated with side effects that are excessively interfering with the patient's quality of life. Having said that, all patients on ongoing epilepsy medication should, in my opinion, as a minimum receive concurrent treatment to protect against the side effects of the medication.

Herbal treatment with the liver-protective milk thistle is an obvious adjunct for these patients. As always, it is important to remember that it's not necessary to choose between holistic treatments and conventional treatments. Epilepsy is a great example of a condition where the two very often go hand-in-hand, to the benefit of the patient.

Apart from the detoxing effect of holistic treatment, such as the liver-protective effect of herbal milk thistle in counteracting the liver-toxic effect of phenobarbitone (the most common epileptic medication), holistic treatments can also address the deeper-lying problem of the nervous system.

Acupuncture has become well established as an adjunctive treatment for epilepsy. The effect varies, but it is well worth a try.

Homeopathy can be invaluable, especially when there are clear patterns or triggers for the seizures, or when the cause is known or suspected. The most common example of this is the situation in which seizures occur for the first time soon after vaccination. This situation should always be treated with the homeopathic remedy Thuja 200C (see pages 49 and 129 on the use of Thuja). Likewise, Nux vom may be used to treat seizures occurring after poisoning, and Natrum sulphuricum (Nat sulph) or Arnica may cure seizures caused by a physical trauma, as after a fall or traffic accident.

Not all seizures can be controlled through treatment, be it with acupuncture, homeopathy, herbs or conventional medication. This is partly due to the fact that seizures are just a symptom, and, in some patients, will be caused by brain tumours or other serious, possibly incurable, undiagnosed disease.

Uncomplicated epilepsy, however, is not, as a rule, a hindrance to a good life, once the right level of medication has been achieved, and carers become used to their animal having the occasional fit.

THE LOCOMOTOR SYSTEM

The locomotor system includes bones, muscles, tendons, and ligaments – in short, all of the body parts that allow us to move. It is also referred to as the musculoskeletal system.

Dogs are more prone to diseases of the musculoskeletal system than cats, for whom these problems are far less common

and, even when present, often don't require treatment.

This has been the traditional viewpoint, at least. In recent years, we have become increasingly aware that we must be careful not to overlook possible painful conditions in the elderly and inactive cat who stops jumping and climbing in favour of a more sedate lifestyle.

Musculoskeletal problems range from innocuous acute strains and injuries to debilitating chronic disease.

SPRAINS AND STRAINS

Any animal can become hurt: the puppy who takes a playful tumble; the active dog who forces a sharp turn at high speed during agility training, and the cat who misjudges a leap.

If your animal is suddenly lame, is walking reluctantly or stiffly, or is noticeably less active than usual, it is always important to have him examined by your vet. Your dog or cat can't tell you where it hurts – or how much. Don't assume that it will pass. Get it checked.

After your visit, if your vet has been unable to find a specific cause of pain but has ruled out serious injury or disease (or perhaps found a sore muscle or joint that just needs time and rest to heal), there are several steps you can take to promote healing.

Your vet may have prescribed short-term painkilling medication, or you may have agreed simply to give it rest and observe for a few days. In either case, once more serious injury has been ruled out, you absolutely should begin holistic supportive treatments too.

A quick and easy first step is to turn to the acute injury remedies in your homeopathic first aid kit. If you know that your dog or cat has been badly bruised (maybe you saw them fall), the homeopathic remedy Arnica 30C or Arnica 200C is always the first thing to give.

In the case of smaller sprains or strains, the remedy mix RRA will often be the most optimal approach. RRA consists of three homeopathic first aid remedies that, together, cover all the relevant tissue damage from strains and sprains of muscles or joints. You'll be surprised at how often it comes in handy.

If your first aid remedies don't seem to be making a visible difference after a few days, contact an holistic vet for more specific advice on the use of homeopathy, acupuncture, or osteopathy in your situation.

Homeopathy for acute sprains and strains

- *All acute injury (bruising): Arnica*
- *Particularly injury to muscle: Rhus toxicodendron (Rhus tox)*
- *Particularly injury to joint capsule, tendons and ligaments: Ruta graveolens (Ruta grav)*

These three homeopathic remedies complement each other extremely well. This is one of very few situations in which it is appropriate to mix several homeopathic remedies together. RRA (Rhus tox, Ruta and Arnica) will aid many different locomotor problems where the above-mentioned tissues need support. RRA 6C given two to three times daily for a few weeks, or until all symptoms have gone, will often make a marked difference in recovery, and will certainly never hurt to use

FRACTURES

Your vet will stabilise and immobilise the fracture and prescribe painkilling medication. On top of this, there are easy steps you can take to support healing and aid recovery.

The homeopathic remedy Arnica belongs in every first aid kit, and should always be given to anyone sustaining a serious physical trauma. It will promote healing in the acute phase as well as help with long-term

complications after trauma. The earlier it is given, the better.

The homeopathic remedy Symphytum specifically promotes the formation of bone callus, and thereby helps broken bones heal. It can cure problematic non-healing fractures, and it may also be given preventatively to anyone with a fracture (even though it has not become a non-healing one), provided it has first been properly stabilised. Unlike Arnica, which can be given within seconds of an accident, Symphytum must be given with more care, and never until the injury has been X-rayed and immobilised. We don't want to speed up bone healing if the bone has not been fully aligned.

Manual treatments such as massage, physiotherapy and osteopathy are always needed during the recovery phase after serious physical injury. It is important to ensure a return to a normal pattern of movement if we are to avoid future problems from muscular tension, uneven gait, and, in the worst case, long-term overload injuries such as osteoarthritis.

CRUCIATE LIGAMENT RUPTURE

The cruciate ligaments run like crossed strings at the front and back of the knee, where their role is to keep the knee from overextending during movement. When injury occurs in the form of tears in or rupture of a cruciate ligament – most often the one on the front of the knee (the anterior cruciate ligament) – the knee will become loose and move around too much, which will eventually lead to injury of the menisci, and ultimately to osteoarthritis.

Cruciate ligament damage is frequently seen in dogs as well as in humans, where it is a common football injury. It is without comparison the most common knee problem in dogs. Still, it can be difficult to make the exact diagnosis without a scan, which is why any dog with knee pain and hind leg lameness

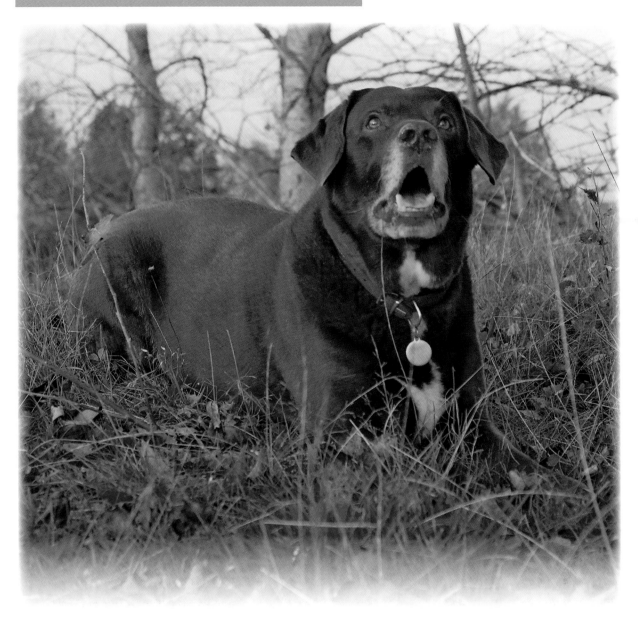

is likely to be referred to an orthopaedic specialist for assessment, and possibly a scan.

This a not a situation where you can afford to wait and see if it clears up by itself, while the unsupported knee sustains further damage that ultimately makes a permanent cure far less likely.

Cruciate problems in dogs may happen, as they generally do in humans: as a sudden, traumatic incident in an otherwise healthy knee joint, typically as a result of a bad fall or a road traffic accident.

There is also another common presentation of cruciate disease in dogs, however, in which the cause of the problem isn't forceful trauma to the knee, but rather a ligament that was weak to begin with. In these cases, the onset of lameness may be gradual, and there will be no report of dramatic injury to the knee. The problem simply gradually worsens over time as the ligament damage progresses, and the knee becomes increasingly inflamed and unstable. In some cases, osteoarthritis is already present in the knee by the time the dog is clearly lame and the problem is diagnosed: a sign that the knee has been unstable for some time.

In a dog who is predisposed to this more chronic form of degenerative cruciate ligament disease, we often see the rather frustrating scenario in which he undergoes surgery on one hind leg, followed by two to three months of rehabilitation, only to then go lame in the other hind leg as the disease becomes noticeable in the opposite knee.

Treatment of cruciate ligament disease

A ruptured cruciate ligament can be surgically repaired (or, to be more precise, a new one can be surgically constructed) via fairly routine knee surgery. This is, however, not always necessary. A rule of thumb says that cruciate-repair surgery is often avoidable in patients weighing less than 10kg. This means that cats and small dogs often recover well with conservative management: in this case rest, painkillers, and physiotherapy.

Large dogs will do best with surgery. The risk of not operating, or of operating too late, is that continued use of the knee by a heavy animal will lead to damage of the menisci, and later to osteoarthritis. The good news is that dogs of all sizes generally do well and regain full use of their knee without long-term complications after appropriate and timely treatment. This absolutely is a problem with a solution.

Holistic treatment of cruciate ligament disease

Regardless of whether your animal is managed conservatively, or needs surgery for his cruciate ligament disease, there are some obvious supportive steps that can help reduce pain, promote healing and support

rehabilitation, making a big difference in his recovery.

The homeopathic remedy RRA 6C, given a couple of times a day for several weeks, will support the structures of the knee. See page 130.

When a dramatic accident was not the reason for ligament damage, and the cause is thought to be an inbuilt tendency to ligament weakness, individual homeopathic treatment can help address this with the aim of preventing a recurrence of the problem in the other knee. If no veterinary specialist homeopath is available, either Ruta grav 30C or Calc phos 30C may be helpful.

Acupuncture is a powerful pain-relieving and anti-inflammatory treatment that is invaluable during all stages of cruciate disease, from painful acute traumatic injury to a case of osteoarthritis following a neglected cruciate ligament rupture.

Manual treatments such as massage, physiotherapy and osteopathy are invaluable during the process of rehabilitation to ensure a full recovery. This is true, whether or not surgery is judged necessary.

Finally, your vet will probably recommend the long-term use of dietary supplements to support regeneration of joint cartilage and joint fluid, and to reduce the risk of developing and severity of osteoarthritis. The most relevant supplements are fish oil and glucosamine. These are given long term; preferably for the rest of the animal's life. See the sections on manual techniques on page 109and supplements on page 212. For a discussion of osteoarthritis (a possible consequence of cruciate disease), see page 197.

DYSPLASIA

Dysplasia is a Greek word meaning 'malformed.' In this context, it is used to describe the integrity of joints.

A joint is a complicated structure where two or more bones meet. It is a very sensitive area in the development of the growing body. If a joint doesn't come together in a harmonious way, it will become unstable, leading to inflammation, pain, and, ultimately, chronic joint disease.

In principle, any joint can develop poorly, but most problems are seen in hips, elbows and shoulders. The bigger the animal, the more growing there is to do, and the greater the risk of joint problems.

The following discussion focuses on hip dysplasia, but the same principles apply to dysplasia of any joint.

Hip dysplasia

Who gets hip dysplasia?
Hip dysplasia is rare in cats and in small dog breeds, and is most commonly seen in large dog breeds such as Golden and Labrador Retrievers, German Shepherds, Rottweilers, Bernese Mountain Dogs, Saint Bernards, and Great Danes.

What is hip dysplasia?
Hip dysplasia means that the hip joint, where the head of the femur (thigh bone) sits in the socket of the hip, is misshapen. This affects the mobility of the joint, and movement of the malformed joint causes continual stress and damage within the joint, which will eventually cause pain and lameness. It typically shows itself in two age groups: the growing puppy and the middle-aged, arthritic dog.

The growing puppy
Some puppies whose hips are malformed will already feel pain during growth, typically at the age of five to ten months. Depending on the severity of the malformation, the pain may subside once the dog is fully grown, and not be felt again until he is middle-aged, and arthritis from walking on an unstable joint becomes evident.

The older dog
The other common presentation is the older dog who is becoming increasingly stiff and unwilling to move.

Arthritis develops as a consequence of a lifetime's movement on malformed hips. Often, this is not noticeable until secondary arthritic changes begin to cause pain, but, upon careful questioning (of the human companion), it sometimes transpires that many of these dogs did have a period of lameness as growing pups, as described above.

Why does a dog develop hip dysplasia?
Hip dysplasia is an hereditary developmental disease in which the hip joint fails to develop properly.

This means that, for a dog to develop hip dysplasia, there must be a genetic predisposition – this is why breeders focus so much on 'hip scores.'

For many generations now, kennel clubs around the world have ensured that only dogs with healthy hips are selected for breeding. It seems a reasonable question, then, to ask why hip dysplasia remains such a common problem.

A case of nature and nurture
Hip dysplasia in dogs remains a very common problem, even after many generations of selective breeding, because genetics is only a part (and maybe even quite a small part) of the problem.

This is a true multifactorial disease, meaning that, in each case, several unfortunate factors come together to result in dysplasia. Some of these factors are known (genetic predisposition, overexercise, overfeeding), some are just being discovered (neutering), and some are probably still not suspected at all.

Puppies are not born with hip dysplasia, but puppies who are genetically predisposed may develop hip dysplasia to varying degrees.

Whether this happens, and to what degree the hips become malformed, is also influenced by factors other than genetics: so-called environmental factors. Research in this area is ongoing, but the advice so far is to avoid overfeeding puppies of large breeds, as too-rapid growth may have a negative effect on hip development in a predisposed puppy.

Avoiding excessive strain on the developing joints by preventing the puppy from using stairs, jumping, standing on his hind legs or being encouraged to run more than he would normally do are all steps than can make an important difference to hip development in the predisposed puppy. This is why puppies (especially of large breeds) should not start activities such as agility or running with their owners until they are fully grown – at least 12 months old.

It is tempting to want to 'tire out' an active eight-month-old dog through jogging, ball throwing or other vigorous activity, but this is absolutely not the way to secure an evening of peace from your teenage dog. You cannot make him tired in this way without putting undue and harmful strain on his skeletal development. Instead, exercise his mind and his nose. Training tricks, following a scent trail and finding hidden objects, people or treats will all keep him stimulated, and help him burn off some of that restless teenage energy. Never try to run him tired.

Recent studies have shown that a puppyhood lifestyle that is too sedentary and restricted in physical activity actually *increases* the risk of hip dysplasia, however. As in all things, we need to strike the right balance: limit inappropriate and harmful strain on the developing joints, but encourage healthy muscle development. These steps seem to make the biggest statistical difference during the first three months of life. Researchers suggest that puppies who have grown up on a farm or had access to a big garden to explore with their littermates are less likely to develop hip dysplasia than those who are kept in more confined conditions, and are therefore less active for the first three months of life.

This is also believed to explain why puppies born in Scandinavia during spring and summer develop fewer hip problems than puppies born in winter, who may not get the same outdoor access during the early months of their lives.

The best way to support healthy hip development in your large-breed puppy is to let him control his activity. Don't take him on long lead walks, don't throw balls or sticks, don't encourage 'clumsy' movements like jumping up on things or climbing stairs, but do let him play freely with other puppies on a daily basis. Go to the park or invite other dog playmates into your garden. Puppies will play actively, giving it all they've got, but they are also good at taking the breaks they need when they are free to do so.

At the time of writing, another important risk factor has emerged which is still news to many. It turns out that neutering is a major risk factor for dysplasia.

See more on this in the chapter about neutering on page 76.

Dysplasia and osteoarthritis: what's the connection?

Hip dysplasia often presents in two distinct age groups, as described above. There is the growing puppy, typically five to ten months old, who experiences pain during the growth phase, and there is the adult, often middle-aged or elderly dog, who has developed osteoarthritis as a consequence of a life of walking on an unstable joint. Osteoarthritis, therefore, is a consequence of dysplasia.

Treatment of dysplasia

Prevention is always better than cure. If you are reading this because you are planning to get a puppy of a large or giant breed that is known to have a high incidence of hip dysplasia, you can certainly reduce the risk of ending up with a dog with hip dysplasia if you follow the advice given here.

Choose a puppy who has parents with good 'hip scores,' and who spends his first few months playing with his littermates in spacious surroundings with outdoor access. Avoid overexercise and overfeeding; let him run free in the park every day, and don't have him neutered.

If you are reading this because your six-month-old puppy has just been to the vet because he has a limp, and you have been told that he has 'loose hips' and to expect problems, don't despair.

Finally, you may have a middle-aged dog who has been diagnosed with hip dysplasia. At this stage, the diagnosis probably actually means that your dog now has osteoarthritis of the hips, because his poorly-formed hip joints are now suffering the consequences.

The symptoms of dysplasia vary from a short period of discomfort in the growing dog to chronic painful and crippling disease. This means, of course, that the need for treatment and the type of treatment varies enormously too. The main message is this: don't despair when you first hear the diagnosis. It is never a hopeless situation, and no dog needs to suffer pain. Much can be done to both protect the joint by slowing the ongoing destruction, and to treat the pain.

The pain may initially be only a phase as the young dog's skeleton matures. After this, many mild or moderate cases will show no signs of discomfort for several years, until osteoarthritis begins to cause problems. The vast majority of dogs diagnosed with hip dysplasia can be helped to lead full lives free of pain. They should not, of course, be used for breeding.

Preventing hip dysplasia

- Choose a puppy from parents with healthy hips. For some breeds, the Kennel Club breeding schemes allow breeding only from parents who have passed a 'hip score' test. Be aware that when purebred puppies are sold without Kennel Club papers, this is sometimes because the parents failed such a test
- Avoid overfeeding your puppy. Youngsters should be lean
- Avoid excessive exercise during his first year. Limit his use of stairs and steps. Discourage jumping and standing on hind legs. Avoid ball or stick throwing. Don't take him jogging or bicycling
- Allow free play to encourage muscle development. Let him run free and play with other puppies
- Don't neuter your dog unless there is a particular reason to do so. Neutering increases the risk of dysplasia

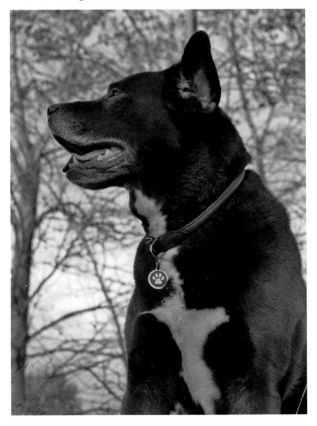

In serious cases of early diagnosed dysplasia, surgery may be needed to establish a working joint. For the vast majority, surgery will not be indicated, and treatment will focus on alleviating pain and, most of all, reducing the development of osteoarthritis in the unstable joint. Avoid obesity. Avoid overexercising, and avoid movements connected with ball or stick throwing, as explained above.

Supplements (especially fish oils, glucosamines, and possibly green-lipped mussels) should be given long term. Osteopathy and physiotherapy can help your dog achieve a natural gait, and acupuncture and massage can help reduce pain, thereby decreasing or removing the need for pain medication. See more in the following section on osteoarthritis.

OSTEOARTHRITIS

Osteoarthritis is far more commonly diagnosed in dogs than in cats. The following therefore refers to dogs, although applies equally to cats.

Why does a dog develop osteoarthritis?

As described in the previous section, osteoarthritis often develops as a consequence of dysplasia. Animals thus affected were born with this tendency, and their joints were always unbalanced.

After several years of use, injury to the joint structures causes enough inflammation and destruction for pain to become a problem.

Osteoarthritis can also, however, be a consequence of traumatic injury that causes chronic joint inflammation. Cruciate ligament injury may cause arthritis of the affected knee years later, and fractures or other traumas due to falls or traffic accidents often lead, as an unavoidable sequela, to osteoarthritis of the affected joints.

Osteoarthritis may also develop as a result of overuse, as seen in sporting dogs or in the very overweight. Finally, it can, to some extent, be seen as a normal sign of aging, as the wear and tear of a long life begin to show.

A wide spectrum

This condition comes in so many forms that it makes sense to categorise patients according to the stage of their arthritis.

The first group consists of dogs who have no symptoms of arthritis, but are judged to be at risk of developing the condition. They may be seen as likely candidates for future problems because their history includes cruciate ligament damage, other trauma or joint surgery. Maybe X-rays have revealed a degree of dysplasia in hips or elbows. Maybe the patients are simply very elderly or belong to heavy breeds. Dogs in this group have no need for pain relief; the aim here is to prevent or delay the development of arthritis.

The second group has already developed mild to moderate degenerative joint disease. These dogs need help repairing the existing damage and preventing further escalation of the problem.

The third group consists of dogs who already suffer pain and decreased mobility. They will show signs of pain, whether through slowing down, becoming more reluctant to move, or presenting lameness or stiffness. These dogs naturally still need help in slowing the rate of inflammatory changes in the joint, but also need effective pain relief and help in avoiding secondary tension from an altered gait.

Treatment of osteoarthritis

Treatment is based on the same principles, regardless of whether we are talking about arthritis of hips, shoulders, elbows, knees or spine.

This is an area of intensive research and development in recent years. Gone are the days when a dog diagnosed with arthritis would be treated solely with ongoing painkilling medication. Today, an array of treatment options exist to ensure maximum benefit and minimum use of drugs (with the inherent risk of side effects after long-term use). Depending on the stage of the disease in each dog, these treatments, when employed, can make a significant difference in quality of life; often for many years.

For the first of the groups described above, the at-risk dogs, the objective is to protect against osteoarthritis developing in the future. The aim is to retain and support the integrity of their joint cartilage and joint fluid in order to keep the joint healthy. This is done primarily through nutraceuticals (food supplements) such as fish oils, glucosamine, chondroitin, and green-lipped mussels. These supplements reduce inflammation of the joint and aid ongoing repair of micro damage to joint structures. The supplements are added to food on a daily, long-term basis.

Apart from supplements, it is important to avoid excessive strain by keeping the dog slim, and not allowing exercise that is too strenuous or excessive. Ball- or stick-throwing games are a bad idea for a dog at risk of arthritis. Swimming is an excellent form of low-impact exercise that strengthens muscles without straining joints. See page 212 for further information about supplements.

The second group, dogs with mild arthritic changes and symptoms, will, in addition to the steps described above (supplements, weight control and exercise caution), also need some kind of regular manipulative therapy. A veterinarian with postgraduate training in osteopathy can help your dog maintain an appropriate gait, which will reduce muscle tension and help prevent the vicious circle of tension leading to pain leading to more tension.

Once the patient starts to favour one joint or limb, the entire gait is altered, and secondary strain and tension are unavoidable.

Using some form of qualified manipulative therapy – be it massage, physiotherapy, chiropractic or osteopathy – is invaluable for these patients, and can sometimes significantly postpone or reduce the need for painkilling medication. Your practitioner may be able to teach you exercises or massage techniques to use at home to strengthen muscles, reduce tension, and support normal body movement. See page 109 for further information on manipulative therapies and page 215 on where to find a qualified practitioner.

Eventually, many arthritic animals will reach the third stage, in which the disease has progressed to a point where they experience pain and significantly reduced mobility. These dogs will naturally still benefit from supplements and manipulative therapies, but they also need pain relief to ensure an optimal quality of life and freedom from pain. Either acupuncture or gold implants will often effectively relieve the pain associated with osteoarthritis. Individually selected homeopathic remedies can also be very helpful in some patients. See page 106 for further information on acupuncture and gold implants, and page 117 on homeopathy.

Even when all of the above measures are used, some dogs will eventually need conventional painkilling medication. If you start with supplements, weight control and exercise restriction, and, when pain becomes evident, move on to manipulative therapies, acupuncture, homeopathy and/or gold implants, you will be able to greatly postpone and reduce the need for painkilling medication. That doesn't mean that it will always be completely avoidable – pain must always be relieved – but there are many steps to take before resorting to long-term medication, with its risk of associated side effects.

There are a vast number of painkilling drugs available, and no one-size-fits-all medication regimen. Together with your vet,

Steps for treating arthritis

- *Nutraceuticals (fish oil, glucosamines, green-lipped mussels)*
  - *Weight restriction*
- *Swimming and other suitable physical activity*
- *Osteopathy/chiropractic/physiotherapy/ massage*
- *Acupuncture (possibly gold implants)*
  - *Homeopathy*
  - *Painkilling drugs*

The above list can, to some extent, be seen as a ladder. Start at the top for the at-risk patient and work your way down the list, adding treatments as the condition becomes more severe

you will determine what drug or combination of drugs has the best effect and is tolerated best by your dog. Be prepared to experiment. Your vet will recommend a blood test before and at regular intervals during treatment to check your dog's liver and kidney function, and ensure that the drugs continue to be well tolerated. You may need a referral to an orthopaedic specialist to get it right. Remember, no one should suffer pain, and there will be a way to relieve pain for every arthritic patient.

SURGERY

The following advice will help you support your animal before and after surgical procedures. It should be regarded as an adjunct to your vet's recommended treatments. If complications

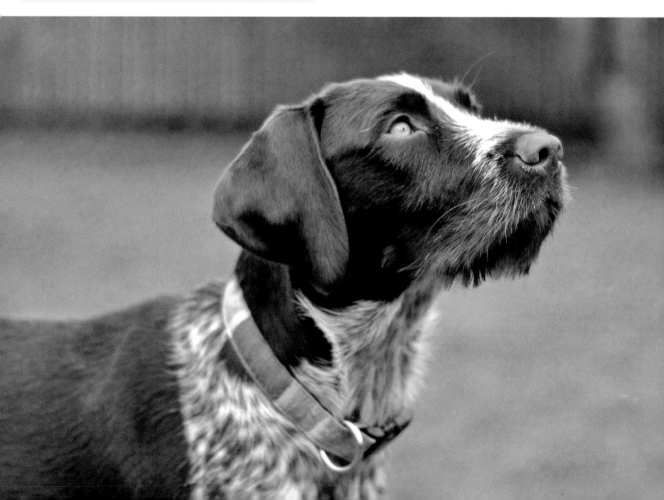

occur, always consult your vet before attempting any home treatment.

The homeopathic remedy Arnica is indispensable in any first aid kit. It is the one supportive step that no surgical patient should ever be without. Arnica is the first remedy to think of when there is physical trauma. If anyone gets hurt, give them Arnica; this applies to humans and animals alike. From the smallest bruise or sprain to the most serious traffic accident or surgical procedure, Arnica will aid recovery.

I always recommend the use of Arnica around dental procedures, neutering, lump removal, or any other surgical procedure, large or small. Give a dose the day before and a dose on the morning of the procedure. Repeat as needed afterwards. You cannot overdose Arnica in cases of physical trauma. Typically, give at least four doses per day for the first few days, tapering off and continuing one or two daily doses until healing is complete, typically after ten to 14 days.

The homeopathic remedy Calendula 30 is indicated when skin or mucous membranes are inflamed. I rarely use it preventatively around general surgery, but highly recommend using it if the surgical wound becomes infected, is very inflamed, or if stitches break down. This may happen as an allergic reaction to the suture material or if your dog or cat manages to lick or scratch the wound. I also recommend Calendula for patients who have had a urinary catheter or surgery involving the bladder. Give one or two daily doses, interspersed with Arnica, as described above.

After spaying, castration or other surgery involving sexual or urinary organs, a single dose (or a couple of doses given on subsequent days) of the homeopathic remedy Staphysagria 200C, given after a couple of weeks, may help prevent long-term imbalances.

In connection with orthopaedic surgery, such as fracture repairs, cruciate-ligament

Arnica

Anyone undergoing a surgical procedure will benefit from the use of the homeopathic remedy Arnica. Use Arnica 30 or Arnica 200. Give one dose the night before and repeat in the morning before going in for the procedure (this does not clash with any instruction to fast).

When you pick up your dog or cat after the procedure, give a dose every one to two hours for the rest of the day, slowly decreasing over the following days from four daily doses to one daily dose. Stop when healing is complete, normally after around ten days. You cannot overdose in this situation. The principle is to match the need. While the trauma is fresh and extensive, treat frequently, and, as healing progresses, taper off. If you are using Arnica for yourself or a human friend, simply take a dose whenever it hurts. This way, you will automatically match the intensity of the symptoms and thereby dose exactly as required. Always have Arnica available at home in case of injury to humans or animals

repairs, treatment of prolapsed discs or anything else to do with the locomotor system, it is crucial to ensure proper rehabilitation. Physiotherapy should always be a part of the support after such procedures in order to ensure that normal gait is restored. This will reduce the risk of secondary tensions and abnormal strain that could otherwise lead to osteoarthritis. Ideally, before recovery is complete have your dog checked by a vet who specialises in osteopathy.

If wound healing is poor or scars cause problems, acupuncture or homeopathy can help.

Physical symptoms or behavioural changes that occur after surgery are best addressed by consulting an experienced homeopath. You may also, if appropriate, see whether you can address behavioural changes yourself by using Bach flower remedies.

BEHAVIOURAL PROBLEMS

Dogs die from lack of socialisation
More dogs are put to sleep because of behavioural problems than for any other reason.

Take a moment to think about that.

Physically healthy animals are euthanised in large number because they are unable to cope. They cannot fit in. They cannot interact peacefully with us or with other dogs, so they are killed. This is all the more tragic because it is entirely preventable.

The good news
That this is entirely preventable is also the good news. So, let's prevent it.

No more puppy farms – buy your new puppy from a home breeder who eagerly answers your questions about socialisation, and explains how she exposes puppies to a vast range of experiences. Take your young puppy out into the world as soon as he comes home with you. You don't want to overwhelm or scare him, but you do want to fill his head with new experiences.

And absolutely no more talk of isolating puppies until after the puppy vaccines. The last puppy vaccine is given at 16 weeks (unless you use titre testing; see page 52), which is precisely when the 'window' closes and puppy socialisation becomes too late. The risk of an unvaccinated puppy catching a potentially fatal contagious disease is endlessly smaller than the risk of a potentially fatal behavioural problem arising from lack of socialisation. Puppies need to get out into the world and learn how to interact and not to be fearful. Missing out on this is the single biggest risk not only to their (and your) quality of life, but also to their longevity.

Poorly-socialised puppies turn into problem dogs
Socialisation means to purposefully expose a puppy to a wide variety of experiences at the appropriate time, and appropriate here means early.

If you adopt a young dog who has spent the first four months of his life in a kennel, he will likely grow into an adult dog who is less confident, flexible, sociable, and able to adapt than the puppy who moves into your home at eight weeks, having spent the first two months of his life with a breeder who understands early socialisation, and has already introduced the puppy to noise, movement, hoovering, people of all ages, and interactions of all sorts.

Between the ages of three weeks and three to four months, a dog's brain is malleable, and primed to learn that new sounds, sights and experiences are nothing to be feared. This is when he learns about relating both to humans and to other dogs. After this period, everything becomes much, much harder, and unknown sights, sounds and experiences are likely to frighten him.

What this means is that the biggest threat to a dog's life is not a horrible, contagious disease. The biggest threats to your puppy living a long and happy life are behavioural problems caused by lack of early socialisation.

The key word here is early. It turns out that it actually is difficult to teach old dogs new tricks. See page 11 on the important puppyhood period.

Puppy classes
I sometimes come across people who send their dog to be trained elsewhere. To my mind, this approach results from a misunderstanding.

Good dog training is a learning process for the human at least as much as for the dog. Dog training is really about the two of you bonding, having fun together, and learning how to trust each other and interact in a

The golden period that shapes a dog's mind

Between the ages of 3 weeks and 3-4 months a puppy's mind is open. It is primed for new experiences, and ready to learn about the world. This is a golden period that must not be wasted for it determines how the dog interacts with his surroundings for the rest of his life

positive way. I highly recommend that you sign up for puppy classes together soon after your puppy arrives.

As he matures, there is a huge selection of other classes to try out. I am a great fan of clicker training, but you may prefer nose work, agility, obedience, dog dancing, rally, or one of the many other human-and-dog activities on offer.

All dogs and their people will benefit from some kind of regular class for at least the first two years, and, if you are both enjoying the shared activity, why stop?

Behavioural therapy

Prevention is certainly easier than cure, but this should never be taken to mean that problems can't be solved. If your dog has developed a problem, be it noise sensitivity, home-alone issues, aversion to car rides, general reactivity, fear or even aggression toward people or dogs, chances are it can be solved if you are willing to make the effort.

It is, however, unlikely that you can solve it alone. Get professional help; the sooner the better. A professional dog behaviourist will prove invaluable as you set out to change things, and to support your dog. The behaviourist will observe you with your dog in problematic situations, and will not only be able to identify steps you can take to work toward a long-term resolution, but will also follow your progress over time and be there to offer advice and encouragement.

Ongoing professional support can make all the difference, and it is an excellent investment at any point where you may feel frustrated with your dog. Whether you are looking for someone to meet with you and your puppy to advise on optimal socialisation from day one, someone to help you survive the challenging 'teenage' period that often dominates the end of a dog's first year, or someone to help with an established problem, the sooner you get help, the easier the process will be, and the better the chance of success.

Give yourself and your dog this gift. It will likely secure your happy relationship for the future. Are you struggling? Is your dog proving difficult? Get help.

Psychotropic drugs

There are drugs that can modify behaviour, and these are typically used to treat anxious dogs, or dogs exhibiting a specific undesirable behaviour.

Personally, I find that these drugs are overused. They may have a place (although I remain unconvinced), but this should always be for a limited period, and only as an adjunct to intensive and targeted training under the guidance of an experienced behavioural therapist. Drugs are, at best, a way to aid and reinforce training. Behaviour-modifying drugs are never a solution in themselves, and they must never stand alone.

Supplements and other products

There are a number of natural methods and products aimed at easing anxiety. Thunder shirts, pheromones, aromatherapy, Bach flower remedies, and food supplements (to name but a few) can all help reduce anxiety in the here and now. These can all be valuable during the odd stressful occasion, such as a house move, an evening of fireworks, a big party next door, a veterinary visit or a long journey.

However, if you have an anxious dog, you'll want to look deeper. Targeted training under the guidance of an experienced dog behaviourist will help you and your dog move on, and put the problem behind you. Individualised homeopathic treatment can help facilitate this process.

The main point here is that change is a process, often even a valuable one, but there is no quick fix. See more about supplements and pheromones on page 214, Rescue Remedy on page 111, and about homeopathy on page 117.

AGGRESSION

The following text addresses aggression and anxiety mainly in dogs. See page 207 for a discussion of common behavioural problems in cats.

Preventing aggressive behaviour

Taking on a puppy means taking on full responsibility for a sensitive and intelligent fellow being for the next ten to 15 years – his whole life. This involves an obligation to become informed about his needs, and, without a doubt, the first and most important need is early and appropriate socialisation.

A puppy who is afforded the time, company and interest of his humans, and who is taken out into the world from a very early age to meet all kinds of people and animals, will learn to interact without problems.

Ten-month-old puppy going cheap?

Most dogs will go through a teenage period, which may be an ordeal for their carers, and even make them question the whole 'let's get a dog' idea (whose idea was that, anyway?). It helps to remember that, as with humans at that age, it is just a phase.

With a good dog trainer on hand to provide understanding and support, these few months are generally best handled with humour and patience. Hang in there and resist the urge to abandon the entire project, or make extreme decisions or changes such as re-homing or neutering. This is how it's supposed to be for a while between the ages of, say, 7 and 14 months. It will pass on its own, and, when it does, you will suddenly be presented with the no-longer-deaf, responsive and enjoyable adult dog who reflects all the work you have put into his early training and socialisation.

Knowing what to expect makes it easier to be patient and understanding, and simply to laugh off those situations in which all you want to do is turn your back and mutter, 'Never seen that dog before in my life – nothing to do with me.'

Off with his genitals?

Briefly put, the idea that castration (males) or sterilisation (females) somehow has a general calming effect, and makes dogs easier to handle is a *complete myth*. On the contrary, new research indicates that neutering a young dog who has shown signs of being reactive, fearful or aggressive is most likely to make the behaviour worse.

Routine neutering has turned out to be associated with a myriad of health problems, and is, in any case, never the way to achieve better control of an unruly youngster. In

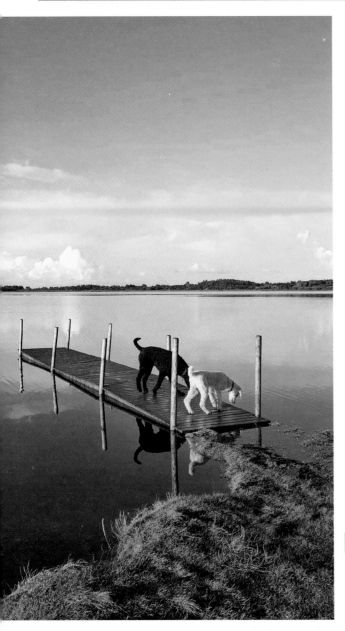

first get your vet to look him over to rule out the possibility that he is ill, and lashing out because of pain. If your vet gives him a clean bill of physical health, the next step is to involve a competent dog behaviourist, who can help you to understand and address the problem in a constructive manner.

Pheromones and supplements can ease stress in both dogs and cats, and can be useful adjuncts in some situations.

Conventional behaviour-modifying drugs may, as previously discussed, play a role in facilitating targeted training under professional guidance. I am sad to say, however, that it is my experience in my daily work that drugs are increasingly seen as an acceptable way to adjust unwanted behaviour in dogs.

I find this overuse of drugs both shocking and inappropriate. What has it come to when we expect our animals to live lives they can cope with only if drugged? Behaviour-modifying drugs are an adjunctive tool to be employed only in the most desperate cases, in which training alone would not suffice, and are never an answer in themselves. They must never stand alone, and they should never be used for more than a couple of months as a way to kickstart long-term training: where the real and permanent changes happen.

ANXIETY

At the significant risk of repeating myself, it must be said that fear, reactivity or anxiety is generally the result of a lack of early socialisation.

We must also not forget that aggressive behaviour, in many cases, is based in fear.

Two very common situations that cause problematic, anxiety-based behaviour in dogs is fear of car rides, and separation anxiety when he is left home alone. These problems vary on a broad scale from slight reluctance to absolute panic. What they have in common is that they are problems with solutions. The

six months, they will have calmed down because they grew up, not because they were neutered.

See also the sections about puppyhood on page 11 and about neutering on page 76.

Dealing with aggressive behaviour

If you have an adult dog who has shown aggression toward other dogs or people, earlier you address the problem, the quicker it will be solved.

Prevention is always easier than cure, but no matter how you got there or how severe your dog's phobia, I promise you that these problems are always solvable. Always.

You will not forever have to arrange your life around needing to take your dog to work with you, employing dog sitters, or taking other measures to avoid these stressful situations, nor will you have to rehome or even euthanise your dog because these issues make your life difficult.

You may need to involve a professional dog behaviourist for a while to guide the process, and you will need to commit to a period of intensive training or 're-learning,' but I promise that it will be worth it.

Fear of car rides or motion sickness

Motion sickness is caused by overstimulation of the labyrinth of the inner ear, that controls balance, resulting in nausea and sometimes vomiting. There is also a significant degree of learned behaviour involved, as someone who is anxious and stressed will be more likely to get carsick. Similarly, someone who has been carsick before may be anxious about getting into the car again

I don't find it very useful to try to distinguish between dogs who suffer true motion sickness, with dizziness and nausea, and those who are agitated 'only' because they fear car rides. No doubt there is a big overlap between the two groups.

All dogs must be able to travel in a car, and all dogs can learn to do so. There are many steps you can take, to both reduce anxiety and relieve nausea. Depending of the nature and severity of the problem, you may choose to use one or more of these. See page 206.

Preventing problems

I suspect that many puppies who develop a strong aversion to car travel were subjected to an unbearable first car ride when they were picked up from the breeder to travel to their new home. If the young puppy experiences being removed from everything he knows to go in a car for the very first time on an hour-long journey, who can blame him if the experience is remembered as a bad one?

There are great breeders who make sure that their puppies are taken on short car rides as part of the early socialisation effort, but, for most puppies, the first car ride will, unfortunately, be associated with what is probably the most stressful day of their lives.

To prevent this becoming a problem, you need to get him, if not straight back on the horse, then straight back into the car in order to turn around his perception. Start by taking him on very short trips. Let him sit on the lap of a passenger, and keep an eye on his reaction. It is okay for him to be slightly worried, but don't let him work himself into a panic. Make sure to stop on a good note, when he is calm.

During the first weeks of his new life with you, try to take him in a car (even if just for five or ten minutes) every day, if possible.

In exactly the same way, training to prevent separation anxiety starts, if not on the first day, then certainly after the first week, when your puppy has settled into his new home. Gradually leave him alone in a room for a few minutes – perhaps while he explores a toy or a tasty treat – while you close the door behind you and hang out the washing, empty the mailbox, or take out the trash. This repeated and brief experience will show him that being alone is temporary and not a big deal.

The next step is to leave him home alone for half-an-hour, making sure to return when he is calm. It is a good idea at this stage to introduce a ritual such as giving him a treat, and saying the same phrase so that he knows what to expect – and then just go. Don't look to him to show you that it's okay. It *is* okay.

Within a month of joining your family, your puppy should be used to being home alone for several hours. In my experience, this happens from necessity in working families, but is easily overlooked or unduly postponed in homes where there is no immediate need for the puppy to be left alone. Whether you are a pensioner, on maternity leave, or working from home when your new puppy moves in, please remember that being alone is a crucial skill that he should learn while he is still very young. See the section on the golden period for socialisation on pages 16 and 202.

Dealing with an established problem

If, for whatever reason, you find that your dog has a real phobia, be it separation anxiety, an aversion to car rides, or an overreaction to a completely different situation or stimulus, turning the negative reaction into a positive one may be a far more involved and demanding process. With daily training, however, it should be possible to see a big shift within a few months.

In these situations, training needs to be broken down into small steps; you never want to ask for more than he is capable of. Never entice or force your reluctant and frightened dog. He needs a small, achievable goal and a reward for reaching it. In this way, step-by-step, milestone-by-milestone, by breaking the impossible and unmanageable into hundreds of small, successful steps, you'll get there in the end. The negative association can and will be turned into a positive one.

I suggest that you turn the training process into a game for both of you. No doubt, you'll get to feel silly along the way. Patience, dedication, and a well-developed sense of humour are the required attributes.

The training (re-learning) starts at the point when your dog begins to show signs of stress. I am going to use car rides in the following example, but the same principle applies to most problems you may need to address. Break the process into many smaller goals, and don't proceed until your dog is completely comfortable with the previous step. Every exercise must end on a positive note.

The benefit of working with a dog behaviourist cannot be overemphasised. Do engage someone who can map out the road, monitor your progress, and support you when you lose heart. This way, the goal is already in sight.

Learning to enjoy car rides (and other overwhelmingly scary experiences)

If your dog begins to look worried as soon as you reach for your car keys or put on your coat, this is precisely where your training starts.

As often as possible every single day, put on your coat and jingle your car keys. Next, put away the keys, disrobe and, with heartfelt excitement, do a joyful victory dance with your dog, preferably involving cheese or whatever treat happens to be his particular favourite. Half-an-hour later, you get to do the whole silly act again.

Once he reacts to you picking up your keys and putting on your coat with happy excitement (or ignores you completely, depending on his temperament) – in other words, once this previous trigger no longer elicits a negative response – you can tick the first box and move on to the next step.

Now, perhaps five times a day, grab your keys, put on your coat, put his leash on him and go halfway down the drive before you (in full view of the neighbours, of course) do your celebration dance, turn around, and go back inside. Before long, you and your dog will cheerfully go and pat the car before he is amply rewarded, and you both go back inside.

Next, you might sit in the car and enjoy a treat before returning inside without ever turning on the engine.

I'm sure you get the picture. It is fun, invariably silly, and requires endless repetition, but it is absolutely doable. Don't look to your dog to assess when he becomes worried and needs to stop. Aim to stop before he becomes worried. Each step may take days or weeks; it takes as long as it takes. Don't ever try to cajole or force him to do something before he is ready. Each negative experience will undermine the process and set you back several steps. For this reason, ideally avoid any car trips at all during the training period. The whole point is to reverse his earlier negative associations; not remind him of them.

Similarly, if what you are addressing is separation anxiety rather than aversion to car rides, you may need to arrange for him never to be home alone for several months until the training is complete.

The above is an outline of a possible training sequence for a dog with a genuine phobia about car rides. If your dog is less affected, you simply start your training at the point where he begins to show unease. The important point is never to start driving with a scared and reluctant dog. We all learn best with fun and rewards. Nobody learns anything from being scared.

Relieving motion sickness
Apart from focused training, as outlined above, there are several things you can try to ease motion sickness. Dogs who suffer carsickness should travel only on an empty stomach. Avoid driving during the heat of the day, and slow down on winding roads. Some dogs prefer being able to look out the window (preferably facing the direction of travel), while others prefer lying on the floor. I'll let you decide whether your dog should travel in a crate, on the front or back seat, but please, please don't let him stick his head out of the window as this can cause inflammation of ears and eyes. If your dog is nervous, a calming food supplement may help.

See page 214 for more on food supplements.

Calming pheromones are available both as a collar and as a spray you can use in the car before setting off. This can make the car a happier place. See page 214 on pheromones.

Ginger has a reputation for settling motion sickness. I have little personal experience of this, but you may wish to give it a try.

Homeopathic medicine works best when chosen specifically for each individual. The following homeopathic remedies are often helpful in cases of severe motion sickness. If you feel like experimenting, you may see a good response from one of these four. Always stick with one remedy at a time.

* Cocculus 30C
* Tabacum 30C
* Petroleum 30C
* Nux vom 30C

If you have tried the advice in this chapter and still have a problem, do see a dog behaviourist. If the problem persists or is obviously physical motion sickness rather than a behavioural issue, seek the advice of a veterinarian who is skilled in classical homeopathy or acupuncture. These issues are always solvable.

BEHAVIOURAL PROBLEMS IN CATS

Stress
Cat owners do, from time to time, seek help because their cat is exhibiting aggressive or fearful behaviour. Much more commonly, however, when I see a cat with a behavioural issue in my clinic, he has been brought to me because stress has led to physical symptoms. It is typically problems of the bladder or skin that raise the alarm (also see the sections on overgrooming, page 164, and idiopathic cystitis, page 179).

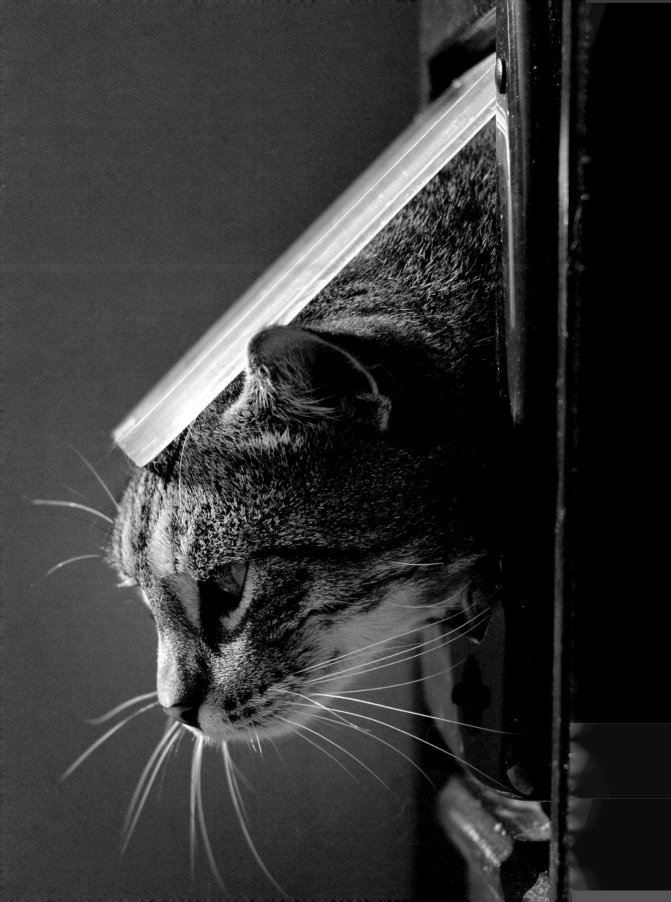

Stressed cats = skin or bladder problems

Cats are (unlike humans, dogs and horses) by nature solitary and independent creatures. No wonder, then, that the living conditions we offer them often lead to stress.

Many cats confined indoors are stressed by the lack of freedom and stimulation. Many cats with outdoor access, particularly in towns and cities, are stressed by the fact that they must share a relatively small territory. In my experience, a very common cause of stress in cats is keeping more than one in the same house, especially during periods of change, such as when a new cat is introduced

Inappropriate urination

If your cat starts peeing outside of the litter box, the first step is to have a urine sample examined to rule out a bladder infection (cystitis) or urinary crystals. If the urine shows no signs of bacteria or crystals, if there are no other signs of physical illness, and if the litterbox is kept clean and in its usual spot with the usual litter, yet your cat is peeing in your bed, on the sofa or on your doormat, then you are likely dealing with a behavioural issue caused by stress.

It can be something of a puzzle to work out what has upset him. Have there been changes in your family life or home? Have you rearranged the furniture? Have you had building work done? Are other cats in the area challenging or bullying your cat? Are they maybe even coming into your house? Has a new cat moved into your home or your area? Have you held parties or had overnight guests? Have you been away on holiday?

A key solution

If your cat is being stressed by other cats coming into his home, the clever solution is to install a cat flap with a key so that only your cat can use it. The older models required your cat to carry a magnet in a collar, but collars and cats are always an extremely bad combination, so it's a big improvement that you can now get a cat flap that reads the cat's microchip. This way, your cat always has an open door if he needs to retreat, and no one else can follow. Surely an elegant solution to a common problem.

Homeopathy

If you believe that your cat is reacting to a perceived insult that explains his peeing in your bed – perhaps your boyfriend moved in, or perhaps the problem started during or just after you went away on a two-week holiday – the homeopathic remedy Staphysagria can often solve the problem (see page 128).

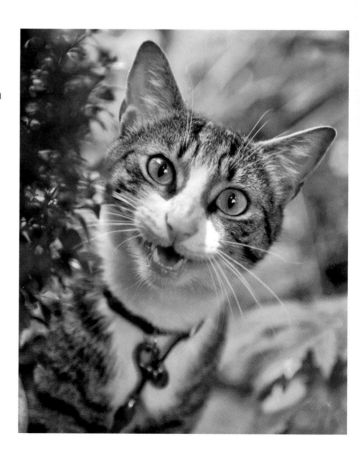

Supplements

Pheromone-based products can often help settle a stressed cat, and can be very useful during periods of change. Food supplements based on tryptophan or colostrum can also have a calming effect on some cats. See page 214.

If none of the above helps, and physical illness has been ruled out, seek the help of a professional cat behaviourist, a veterinary homeopath, or an acupuncturist. If all else fails, regrettably, rehoming your cat to somewhere with outdoor access or without other cats may be the only solution.

Cats and travel

Cats generally don't need to travel by car except for the occasional vet visit, but if you have a cat who gets very stressed by car journeys, spraying a pheromone product into the cage before setting out can be very helpful (see page 214). Rescue Remedy from the Bach flower remedy series has a calming effect in times of stress, but in my opinion it has to be repeated too frequently to be very useful during long trips.

It is a decidedly bad idea to have a stressed cat loose in the car, which is why I advise against administering anything during the trip. This is why applying a pheromone spray in the car is often the most practical method of calming a cat during journeys. If you are going on a very long trip and you know from experience that pheromones alone are not sufficient, talk to your vet about medications. Remember that it is best for your cat to travel on an empty stomach.

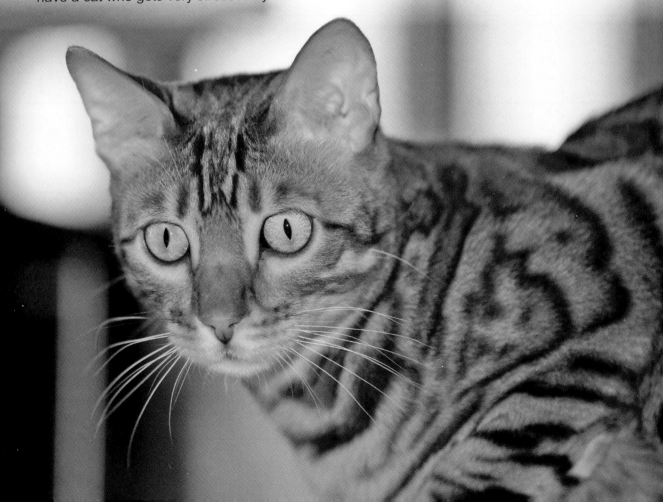

Appendices

Some of my favourite nutraceuticals and other products

This section covers a small number of products that I frequently recommend for my patients. They have little in common, and could just as naturally have been covered, perhaps, in the chapters on herbal medicine or behavioural problems, or under each disease condition. The reason for grouping them together here is purely for ease of reference.

Many years ago, I decided that I would not sell any products in my practice. I sell only professional advice. Over the years, athough some products have proven of great value to certain patients, I continue to not sell or supply these myself, relying instead on my clients purchasing the recommended products elsewhere. I think we should be careful about supplementing on a long-term basis without a clear reason to do so, especially in healthy individuals.

As you have no doubt gathered, I am really not into products, although I understand the temptation to shop for that next cream, snack or supplement for the animal in your life. Most of the time, I prefer that my clients resist the urge: less is more.

I do not and have never received any payment for recommending any product, and I have had no contact with the manufacturers of the products mentioned here.

I stubbornly stick to the principle of not administering anything when there is no known need or benefit. Having said that, the fact remains that there are a few supplements that I frequently recommend, and which I would hate to be without, as they have clearly benefited many of my patients. If, for whatever reason, you have no access to an holistic vet, you should know about these products, too. Truth be told, most of these are now so widespread that most purely conventional veterinary practices will recommend them also.

My minimal list of indispensable supplements looks like this –

Supplements for liver disease
MILK THISTLE

There are at least a handful of veterinary products that contain the active ingredient of herbal milk thistle – silybin – in combination with other liver protectants such as SAMe. Any good local veterinary clinic will be able to supply these and advise about their use.

You may also choose to use the pure herbal tincture of milk thistle, though this option may make it harder to establish the exact concentration of the active ingredient. Make sure to buy such products from a reputable supplier.

Milk thistle is such a potent liver protectant that its use is sometimes recommended as a general detoxing substance: ask your vet for advice. I recommend on-going supplementation with milk thistle (or a product containing its active ingredient, silybin) to dogs and cats receiving medications that are known to put a strain on the liver. Patients on antiepileptic medication are a good example.

Supplements to support the skin
ESSENTIAL FATTY ACIDS (EFA)
Evening primrose oil or a mixture containing it has long been a favourite source of EFA to support healthy skin and coat. EFA supplementation alone will not take away an itch or cure any skin condition, but it is a nice additional support for the skin, and often adds a noticeable shine to the coat.

Supplements for musculoskeletal problems
GLUCOSAMINE AND CHONDROITIN
FISH OIL
GREEN LIPPED MUSSEL EXTRACT
These supplements are given to reduce the inflammation associated with osteoarthritis, and to provide the building blocks needed to repair damaged cartilage and joint fluid.

I find there is great individual variation when it comes to each patient's response. Some arthritic patients experience a marked reduction in pain, whilst others don't seem to respond much, or at all: it's worth experimenting with different products.

To some extent, these supplements are given to halt a process that is constantly worsening, which means that it can be hard to know exactly how much they are helping. A patient with chronic degenerative joint disease who stops deteriorating, or even experiences slowing of the rate of deterioration, is clearly

responding well, even though no immediate *improvement* may be noticed.

I recommend giving one or all of these supplements to all dogs with arthritis, all dogs with prior orthopaedic injuries, or where there are other reasons to suspect that osteoarthritis is likely to develop. You could argue that this is a sensible precaution for all middle-aged dogs of large breeds.

Generally, the supplements are given long-term and on a daily basis.

Supplements for diseases of the urinary system (kidney and bladder)
PHOSPHATE BINDERS (IPAKITINE OR EPIKACIN)
Adding a phosphate binder to the diet reduces the absorption of phosphate from the intestine. Dogs and cats with kidney disease will often be restricted to a high-calorie and low-

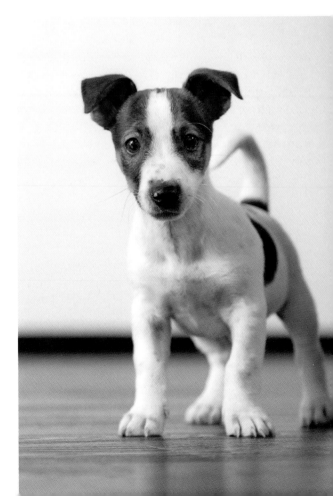

Oils

Essential fatty acids (EFA) play a large role in the health of humans and animals alike. Oils derived from plants and fish oils are both used as supplements:
Fish oils are regarded as particularly beneficial to heart, joints, and nerve tissue (including the brain). This makes fish oil relevant to all heart patients, and to all patients suffering from arthritis. For this reason, fish oil supplementation is probably a good idea for all aging cats and dogs.
Plant oils are regarded as particularly beneficial to hormones, and to the skin and coat. I recommend this supplement to any patient suffering from allergic skin disease.

phosphate diet ('kidney-diet'). One benefit of a phosphate binder is that it frees you from having to stick to a strict low-phosphate kidney diet, which can be a great relief if your animal is not keen on eating the diet your vet has recommended.

Remember that for an animal suffering from kidney disease, eating anything is better than starving because what is on offer is not agreeable to him. See page 184 about kidney disease.

CystoPro

Contains an antioxidant derived from cranberries (proanthocyanidin), together with probiotics and ingredients to soothe the lining of the bladder wall. I find long-term use of this product very valuable in both dogs and cats who suffer recurring bouts of bacterial cystitis.

Cranberries

If your dog suffers from acute cystitis, you may simply choose to feed him fresh or dried cranberries alongside the antibiotics prescribed by your vet. Compared to a

standardised extract, the disadvantage of giving fresh berries is that it is difficult to be sure of the concentration and dosage. There may, on the other hand, be health benefits in giving the complete berries.

Cystophan

Like CystoPro, Cystophan contains ingredients that support the lining of the bladder wall. It also contains the amino acid tryptophan, which has a calming effect on some overly-anxious individuals. For this reason, it is particularly relevant as a supplement for cats who suffer from recurring idiopathic cystitis, as this condition is believed to be stress-related in cats (see page 179).

Supplements for diseases of the digestive system

Probiotics

Probiotics are concentrated batches of 'good bacteria' that are given to help restore an optimal gut flora. There are many situations where this can be helpful.

In acute cases of diarrhoea, probiotics are often given as a paste mixed with a binding agent. This is an excellent first port of call any time your dog has loose stools. Probiotic supplementation is also a great idea after a course of antibiotics, or in any other situation where the natural gut flora may need strengthening.

Probiotics in powder or capsule form can also be given on a more long-term basis if your animal suffers from chronic gastro-intestinal disease. Increasingly, the microbiome (the bacterial make-up of the intestinal tract) is seen as the key to good health in general - not just in relation to digestive health. Following this line of thinking, giving a high-quality probiotic for a few weeks may be a good idea whenever there is a stressful event happening in your animal´s life, be it vaccination, surgery, diet changes, travel, or any other situation where he requires extra support.

SLIPPERY ELM

Slippery elm is a herbal medicine: a tree bark that, upon contact with liquid, forms a slimy gel. The gel has a soothing and lubricating effect on the lining of the gut, and is therefore a very useful supplement to use in cases of both diarrhoea and constipation. It can be used short-term or on an on-going basis.

This is, for example, a very useful supplement for dogs with IBD (inflammatory bowel disease) until a more deep-acting cure can be found.

PSYLLIUM HUSKS

Psyllium husks are a source of natural fibre. They draw liquid from the intestines which makes the husks swell. This can be helpful in cases of both acute diarrhoea and chronic constipation.

Some cats with irreversible megacolon, for instance, benefit from having a small amount of psyllium husks added to their food every day. It is important that patients receiving psyllium husks drink plenty of water. Ask your vet for advice.

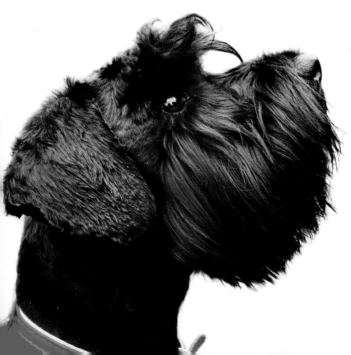

Supplements and other products with an effect on behaviour

PHEROMONES

The pheromones used in Adaptil (for dogs) and Feliway (for cats) are not supplements, but rather airborne compounds that mimic natural dog and cat pheromones, and seem to have a calming effect on many anxious animals. These products are primarily intended to be distributed throughout the home using a plug-in pheromone diffuser. Human noses are not sensitive enough to pick up any scent.

My experience is that they have no effect for some, whilst others swear by them, and feel a distinct change in their animal's behaviour when the diffuser runs out and needs a refill. These pheromones are also available in the form of a spray to use in transport cages, in the car, on the vet's table, or in any other situation that may otherwise seem threatening to your animal.

TRYPTOPHAN

Tryptophan is an amino acid that, in the body, acts as a precursor to the neuro-transmitter serotonin. It is suggested that, by increasing serotonin levels in the brain, tryptophan can help some cases of depression and anxiety. Tryptophan can be found in a wide range of foods, treats and supplements.

CASEIN AND THEANINE

These compounds, derived from milk protein and tea respectively, seem to have calming properties in many anxious dogs and cats. Zylkene and KalmAid are examples of available products.

HERBAL SCULLCAP AND VALERIAN

A herbal mixture commonly used to ease fear and anxiety.

THUNDER SHIRT

A tight wrap that supposedly works similarly to the old practice of calming babies by swaddling them. Some dogs seem to find reassurance from a thunder shirt. Some carers find that a scarf or an old T-shirt can produce the same effect.

The products mentioned here can be used separately or in combination to provide support for animals who are anxious by nature, or those going through stressful experiences. If trying to smooth a stressful event such as a long journey, the introduction of a new animal, a house move or an evening of fireworks, you will probably only be using these for a limited time – maybe even just for a day or two. If, on the other hand, you are attempting to calm a generally anxious dog or cat, they may be required on an on-going basis. In these cases, I strongly recommend that you don't rely on the above suggestions alone, but also involve a dog or cat behaviourist, and possibly an holistic veterinarian.

USEFUL CONTACTS

Associations and other great links to be aware of

The following is a list of veterinary associations and their websites that will help you find a vet in your area who has received further training in holistic treatment. Some associations will focus on a single treatment form, whilst others will have members with a variety of qualifications.

If your area does not have an organisation specifically for the treatment form you need, you may find a practitioner listed under a more general association.

Acupuncture
- American Academy of Veterinary Acupuncture (AAVA) www.aava.org
- Association of British Veterinary Acupuncturists (ABVA) www.abva.co.uk
- Association of Veterinary Acupuncturists of Canada (AVAC) www.avacanada.org
- Australian Veterinary Acupuncture Group (AVAG) www.acuvet.ava.com.au
- Austrian Veterinary Acupuncture Society (AVAS) www.ava-austria.org
- Belgian Veterinary Acupuncture Society (BEVAS) www.bevas.eu
- Brazilian Association of Veterinary Acupuncture www.abravet.com.br
- Chi Institute of Traditional Chinese Veterinary Medicine (TCVM) www.tcvm.com
- Deutchen Gesellschaft fur Veterinar akupunktur www.gervas.org
- International Veterinary Acupuncture Society (IVAS) www.ivas.org
- Ivas Espana www.ivasespana.com
- Samenwerkende Nederlandse Veterinaire Acupuncturisten www.acupunctuurbijdieren.ln
- Nordisk Veterinær Akupunktur Selskab www.novasweb.wordpress.com
- Societa Italiana di Agupuntura Veteriaria (SIAV) www.siav-itvas.org

Diet
- Raw Feeding Veterinary Society (RFVS) www.rfvs.info

Herbal medicine
- The College of Integrative Veterinary Therapies (CIVT) www.civtedu.org
- Veterinary Botanical Medicine Association (VBMA) www.vbma.org

Holistic Veterinary Associations
- American Holistic Veterinary Medical Association (AHVMA) www.ahvma.org
- Complementary Veterinary Medicine Branch New Zealand www.nzva.org.nz/page/cvmb
- Complementary Veterinary Medicine Group (CVMG) www.cvmg.co.za
- Gesellschaft fur Ganzheitliche Tiermedizin (GGTM) www.ggtm.de
- Schweizerische Tierartzliche Vereinigung fur Komplementar- und Alternativmedizin www.camvet.ch

Homeopathy
- Academy of Veterinary Homeopathy (AVH) www.theavh.org
- British Association of Homeopathic Veterinary Surgeons (BAHVS) www.bahvs.com
- International Association for Veterinary Homeopathy (IAVH) www.iavh.org
- Japanese Association of Veterinary Homeopathy (JAVH) www.javh.jp
- Magyar Homeopata Orvosi Egyesulet www.homeopata.hu
- Osterreichische Gesellschaft fur Veterinarmedizinische Homoopathie www.oegvh.at
- Societa Italiana di Omeopatia Veterinaria (SIOV) www.siov.org

Homeopathic pharmacies
- www.ainsworths.com
- www.hahnemannlabs.com
- www.helios.co.uk

Manual therapies
- American Association of Rehabilitation Veterinarians (AARV) www.rehabvets.org
- Association of Animal Osteopaths (note that members are not vets) www.associationofanimalosteopaths.com
- European Veterinary Society for Osteopathy (EVSO) www.evso.eu
- International Veterinary Chiropractic Association (IVCA) www.ivca.de
- The American Veterinary Chiropractic Association www.animalchiropractic.org
- Tierartzliche Akademie fur Osteopathie-equilibre www.tao-equilibre.de

Parasite control
- www.wormcount.com: an independent UK- based laboratory that offers a global faecal screening service to check whether your animal has worms. It accepts samples from both vets and directly from the public

Vaccination
- World Small Animal Veterinary Association (WSAVA) www.wsava.org/Guidelines/Vaccination-Guidelines

REFERENCES AND FURTHER READING

VACCINATION

Articles
- Day, Horzinek, Schultz: WSAVA Guidelines for the Vaccination of Dogs and Cats, Journal of Small Animal practice, vol 51, June 2010
- Day: Isopathic prevention of kennel cough. Is vaccination justified?, International Journal for Homeopathy 1987, vol 2, 45-50
- Dodds: Half-dose CDV and CPV vaccine study in small breed adult dogs. JAHVMA, vol 41, 12-21 2015
- Killey, Mynors, Pearce, Neil, Prentis, Day: Long-lived immunity to canine core vaccine antigens in UK dogs as assessed by an in-practice test kit. Journal of Small Animal Practice 2017
- Lappin et al, Interstitiel nephritis in cats inoculated with Crandell Rees feline kidney cell lysates, Journal of Feline medicine and Surgery (2006) 8, 353-356
- Lund, Prior, Madsen: Testing dogs for immunity against canine parvovirus, canine distemper virus and canine hepatitis
- Schultz et al: Age and long-term protective immunity in dogs and cats. J Comp Path, 2010, vol142, S102-S108
- Scott-Moncrieff et al, Evaluation of antithyreoglobulin antibodies after routine vaccination in pet and research dogs, Journal of American Veterinary Medical Association 2002, vol 221, 515-521

Websites
- World Small Animal Veterinary Association www.wsava.org (expert vaccination guidelines)

- www.aahanet.org
- www.canine-health-concern.org.uk

PARASITES

Articles
- Wood, Goulson: The environmental risks of neonicotinoid pesticides. Environ Sci Pollut Res Int 2017; 24(21): 17285-17325

Websites
- www.wormcount.com

DIET

Articles
- Dunayer Eric: New findings on the effect of xylitol ingestion in dogs, veterinary medicine, December 2006, 791-796

Books
- *Give Your Dog a Bone* – Ian Billinghurst
- *Honey's Natural Feeding Handbook for Dogs* – Jonathan Self
- *Raw Meaty Bones* – Tom Lonsdale
- *The Lucky Dog Weight Loss Plan* – Vicky Marshal

Websites
- www.rfvs.info

NEUTERING

Articles
- Hart et al: Long-term health effects of neutering dogs – Comparison of Labrador Retrievers with Golden Retrievers. 2014
- Hart et al: Neutering of German Shepherd dogs – associated joint disorders, cancers and urinary incontinence. 2016
- Houlihan: A literature review on the welfare implications of gonadectomy of dogs. Journal of Small Animal medicine 2017
- Kim, Yeon, Houpt: Effects of ovariohysterectomy on reactivity in German Shepherd Dogs. Veterinary Journal 2006
- O'Farrell, Peachey: Behavioural effects of ovariohysterectomy on bitches. Journal of Small Animal Practice 1990

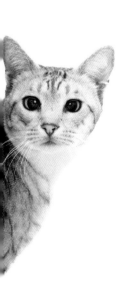
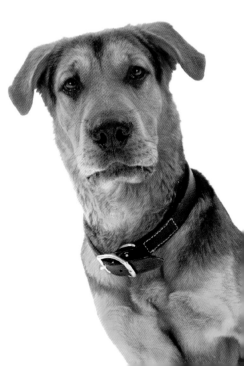

- Sundburg et al: Gonadectomy effects on the risk of immune disorders in the dog: a retrospective study. University of California, Davis, BMC Veterinary Research 2016

- Torres de la Riva et al: 'Neutering dogs: Effects on joint disorders and cancers in Golden Retrievers.' University of California, Davis 2013

- Zink et al: Evaluation of the risk and age of onset of cancer and behavioural disorders in gonadectomized Vizslas. 2014

WEBSITES

- www.avma.org
- www.parsemusfoundation.org/projects/ovary-sparing-spay

HOMEOPATHY

Articles

- Bornhoft, Matthiessen: Homeopathy in Healthcare, effectiveness, appropriateness, safety, cost, Published by Springer-Verlag Berlin Heidelberg New York, 2011
  This report in book form was written by two doctors as part of the Swiss complementary medicine evaluation programme, and is the largest meta-analysis on the effect of homeopathic treatment. It forms the basis on which homeopathy was subsequently included in the Swiss public health care system

- Hill, Hoare, Lau-Gillard, Rybnicek, Mathie: Pilot study of the effect of individualised homeopathy on the pruritus associated with atopic dermatitis in dogs. Veterinary Record (2009) 164, 364-370

- Mathie, Baitson, Hansen, Elliott, Hoare: Homeopathic prescribing for chronic conditions in feline and canine veterinary practice, Homeopathy (2010), 99, 243-248

- Montagnier: Electromagnetic Signals are Produced by Aqueous Nanostructures derived from bacterial DNA sequences, Interdiscip Sci Comput Life Sci (2009) 1, 81-90

Books
- *Homeopathic Care for Cats and Dogs: Small Doses for Small Animals* – Don Hamilton
- *Homeopathy: Medicine for the New Millennium* – George Vithulkas
- *Insights into Veterinary Homeopathy* – Peter Gregory

Websites
- www.ainsworths.com
- www.hahnemannlabs.com
- www.helios.co.uk

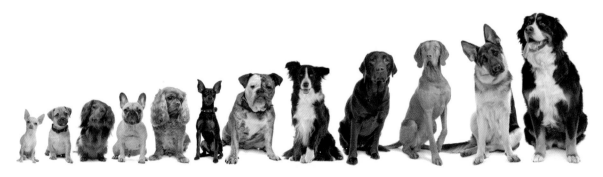

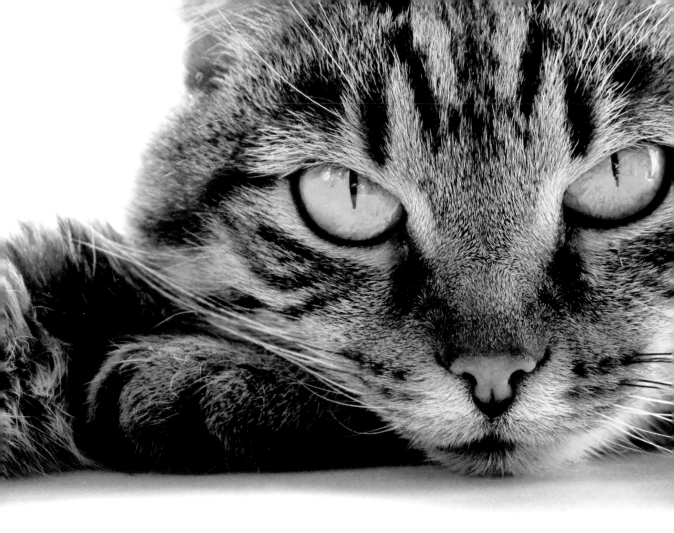

The message that I hope stays with you when you put down this book is the importance of treating each sick animal as an individual. No two allergic dogs are the same, and no two cats with kidney disease will benefit from exactly the same approach. There is no general piece of advice or treatment that will be beneficial to everyone – not even those suffering from the same condition.

This means that important decisions relating to your dog or cat must be made in partnership with your chosen vet.

Don't expect to be able to treat serious illness at home purely on the basis of advice from a book.

I aim simply to inspire both you and your vet to look wider and deeper for the solution that will cure your animal.

Lise Hansen can be contacted at lise@ alternative-vet.co.uk/www.alternative-vet.co.uk

Index

bold indicates main listing for entry

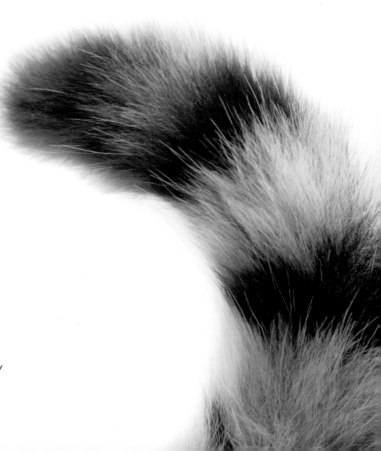

Visit Hubble and Hattie on the web: www.hubbleandhattie.com
hubbleandhattie.blogspot.co.uk
• Details of all books • Special offers • Newsletter • New book news

Also from Hubble & Hattie

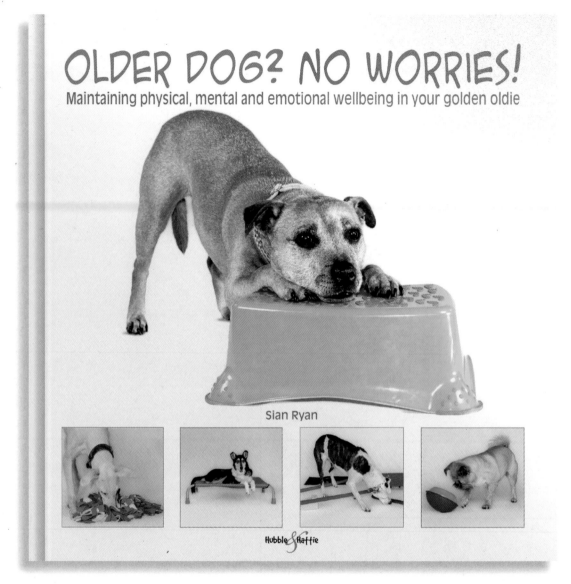

OLDER DOG? NO WORRIES!
Maintaining physical, mental and emotional wellbeing in your golden oldie

Sian Ryan

Hubble & Hattie

Everything you need to know to maximise quality of life for your older dog. Offering advice and ideas for mental, physical, and emotional support as your dog ages and his needs change, including the latest research, and designed to help you create a bespoke care plan for your dog.

Paperback • 96 pages • 100 colour images
• 205x205mm • ISBN 9781787113664 • £13.99*

prices subject to change • p&p extra